DEPRESSIVE DISORDERS

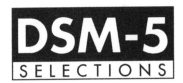

DEPRESSIVE DISORDERS

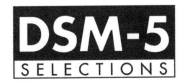

American Psychiatric Association

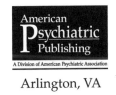

Arlington, VA

Copyright © 2016 American Psychiatric Association

DSM® and DSM-5® are registered trademarks of the American Psychiatric Association. Use of these terms is prohibited without permission of the American Psychiatric Association.

ALL RIGHTS RESERVED. Unless authorized in writing by the APA, no part of this book may be reproduced or used in a manner inconsistent with the APA's copyright. This prohibition applies to unauthorized uses or reproductions in any form, including electronic applications.

Correspondence regarding copyright permissions should be directed to Permissions, American Psychiatric Publishing, 1000 Wilson Boulevard, Suite 1825, Arlington, VA 22209-3901.

Manufactured in the United States of America on acid-free paper.

ISBN 978-1-61537-010-8 (Paperback)

American Psychiatric Association
1000 Wilson Boulevard
Arlington, VA 22209-3901
www.psych.org

Depressive Disorders: DSM-5® Selections is an anthology published by the American Psychiatric Association from the following sources:

American Psychiatric Association: *Diagnostic and Statistical Manual of Mental Disorders*, Fifth Edition. Arlington, VA, American Psychiatric Association, 2013

Black DW, Grant JE: *DSM-5® Guidebook: The Essential Companion to the Diagnostic and Statistical Manual of Mental Disorders, Fifth Edition*. Washington, DC, American Psychiatric Publishing, 2014

Barnhill JW: *DSM-5® Clinical Cases*. Washington, DC, American Psychiatric Publishing, 2014

Muskin PR: *DSM-5® Self-Exam Questions: Test Questions for the Diagnostic Criteria*. Washington, DC, American Psychiatric Publishing, 2014

Contents

Introduction to DSM-5® Selections

Welcome to *DSM-5 Selections*. The purpose of this series is to educate readers about important diagnostic issues associated with categories of DSM-5 disorders. The initial books in the **DSM-5 Selections** series are *Sleep-Wake Disorders, Depressive Disorders, Schizophrenia Spectrum and Other Psychotic Disorders, Feeding and Eating Disorders, Neurodevelopmental Disorders,* and *Anxiety Disorders*. Each book in the series includes the diagnostic criteria relevant to the disorders included in each category. The criteria are taken directly from DSM-5, the most comprehensive, current, and critical resource for clinical practice available today. Also included in each book in the series are extracts from the **DSM-5 Guidebook, DSM-5 Clinical Cases,** and **DSM-5 Self-Exam Questions.** Consequently, each book in the series offers readers a unique introduction to individual categories of DSM-5 disorders and an opportunity to test one's knowledge about DSM-5 disorders.

DSM-5 Guidebook serves as a roadmap to DSM-5 disorders for clinicians and researchers. It illuminates the content of DSM-5 by teaching mental health professionals how to use the revised diagnostic criteria, and it provides practical content for its clinical use. The book offers a fresh perspective to DSM diagnostic categories by focusing on the changes between DSM-IV-TR and DSM-5 that will most significantly impact clinical application of the criteria.

DSM-5 Clinical Cases presents composite patient cases that exemplify the diagnostic criteria for disorders contained in a category. **DSM-5 Clinical Cases** makes DSM-5 come alive for teachers, students, and clinicians. The book helps readers to understand diagnostic concepts, including symptoms, severity, comorbidities, age of onset and development, dimensionality across disorders, and gender and cultural implications.

The questions in **DSM-5 Self-Exam Questions** were written to test readers' knowledge of conceptual changes to DSM-5, specific changes to diagnoses, and the diagnostic criteria. Each question includes short answers that explain the rationale for each correct answer and contain important information on diagnostic classification, criteria sets, diagnoses, codes, severity, culture, age, and gender. The questions are helpful for preparing for various examinations.

The **DSM-5 Selections** series is not intended to replace DSM-5 or the other books from which the extracts are taken. Rather, the series is intended to give readers key selected materials that pertain directly to specific disorder categories. If you find that you require more information about a specific disorder or category of disorders, you are encouraged to examine an APP textbook or clinical manual. You can review the full list of APP titles at www.appi.org.

Robert E. Hales, M.D.
Editor-in-Chief

Preface

Depressive disorders are one of the most common categories of psychiatric disorders. With regard to specific depressive disorders, major depressive disorder has a lifetime prevalence rate of approximately 16% and a 1-month prevalence rate of 6%. DSM-5 includes eight different disorders, each with its own diagnostic criteria. Although major depressive disorder begins with a single episode, 50% of patients will have a recurrence within the first year, and up to 85% will have a recurrence during their lifetime. Major depressive disorders usually last approximately 6 months, with 20% of episodes becoming chronic. There is a higher prevalence of depressive disorders in women. In addition, suicide attempts are also higher in women, but the risk for suicide completion in women is lower.

The possibility of suicidal behavior should be explored with patients who have any of the depressive disorders. Although one of the most commonly described factors is a past history of suicide attempts, most completed suicides are not preceded by attempts. Consequently, it is vitally important for clinicians to conduct a thorough evaluation of the patient with a depressive disorder to rule out suicidal ideation or behavior.

There are many medical diseases that have been associated with depressive disorder, such as cancer, stroke, myocardial infarction, and pregnancy. One of the depressive disorders occurs in childhood (disruptive mood dysregulation disorder), and another is associated with a woman's menstrual cycle (premenstrual dysphoric disorder). Other types of depressive disorders are substance or medication induced or due to another medical condition.

Finally, there are acute and severe episodes of depression such as major depressive disorder and chronic, low-grade disorders characterized by depressive mood for at least 2 years. Heterogeneity of these conditions makes it difficult to make any broad conclusions except that each depressive disorder is associated with depressive symptoms of variable severity.

The changes made to the DSM-5 diagnostic criteria for depressive disorders are highlighted below. This is not meant to be an exhaustive guide to DSM-5 changes, and minor changes in text or wording made for clarity are not described. Section I of DSM-5 contains a full description of changes pertaining to the chapter organization in DSM-5, the multiaxial system, and the introduction of dimensional assessments.

Adapted from McInnis MG, Riba M, Greden JF: "Depressive Disorders," in *The American Psychiatric Publishing Textbook of Psychiatry*, 6th Edition. Edited by Hales RE, Yudofsky SC, Roberts LW. Washington, DC, American Psychiatric Publishing, 2014, pp. 353–389.

Highlights of Changes From DSM-IV-TR to DSM-5

DSM-5 contains several new depressive disorders, including disruptive mood dysregulation disorder and premenstrual dysphoric disorder. To address concerns about potential overdiagnosis and overtreatment of bipolar disorder in children, a new diagnosis, disruptive mood dysregulation disorder, is included for children up to age 18 years who exhibit persistent irritability and frequent episodes of extreme behavioral dyscontrol. On the basis of strong scientific evidence, premenstrual dysphoric disorder has been moved from DSM-IV Appendix B, "Criteria Sets and Axes Provided for Further Study," to the main body of DSM-5. Finally, DSM-5 conceptualizes chronic forms of depression in a somewhat modified way. What was referred to as dysthymia in DSM-IV now falls under the category of persistent depressive disorder, which includes both chronic major depressive disorder and the previous dysthymic disorder. An inability to find scientifically meaningful differences between these two conditions led to their combination with specifiers included to identify different pathways to the diagnosis and to provide continuity with DSM-IV.

Major Depressive Disorder

Neither the core criterion symptoms applied to the diagnosis of major depressive episode nor the requisite duration of at least 2 weeks has changed from DSM-IV. Criterion A for a major depressive episode in DSM-5 is identical to that of DSM-IV, as is the requirement for clinically significant distress or impairment in social, occupational, or other important areas of life, although this is now listed as Criterion B rather than Criterion C. The coexistence within a major depressive episode of at least three manic symptoms (insufficient to satisfy criteria for a manic episode) is now acknowledged by the specifier *with mixed features*. The presence of mixed features in an episode of major depressive disorder increases the likelihood that the illness exists in a bipolar spectrum; however, if the individual concerned has never had symptoms that met criteria for a manic or hypomanic episode, the diagnosis of major depressive disorder is retained.

Bereavement Exclusion

In DSM-IV, there was an exclusion criterion for a major depressive episode that was applied to depressive symptoms lasting less than 2 months following the death of a loved one (i.e., the bereavement exclusion). This exclusion is omitted in DSM-5 for several reasons. The first is to remove the implication that bereavement typically lasts only 2 months, when both physicians and grief counselors recognize that the duration is more commonly 1–2 years. Second, bereavement is recognized as a severe psychosocial stressor that can precipitate a major depressive episode in a vulnerable individual, generally beginning soon after the loss. When major depressive disorder occurs in the context of bereavement, it adds an additional risk for suffering, feelings of worthlessness, suicidal ideation, poorer somatic health, and worse interpersonal and work functioning and an increased risk for persistent complex bereavement disorder, which is now described with explicit criteria in "Conditions for Further Study" in DSM-5 Section III. Third, bereavement-related major depression is most likely to occur in individuals with past personal and family histories of major depressive episodes. It is genetically influenced by and is associated with similar personality characteristics, patterns of comorbidity, and risks of chronicity and/or recurrence as non-bereavement-related major depressive episodes. Finally, the depressive symptoms associated with bereavement-related depression respond to the same psychosocial and medication treatments as non-bereavement-related depression. In the criteria for major depressive disorder, a detailed footnote has replaced the more simplistic DSM-IV exclusion to aid clinicians in making the critical distinction between the symptoms characteristic of bereavement and those of a major depressive episode. Thus, although most people experiencing the loss of a loved one experience bereavement without developing a major depressive episode, evidence does not support the separation of loss of a loved one from other stressors in terms of its likelihood of precipitating a major depressive episode or the relative likelihood that the symptoms will remit spontaneously.

Specifiers for Depressive Disorders

Suicidality represents a critical concern in psychiatry. Thus, the clinician is given guidance on assessment of suicidal thinking or plans and the presence of other risk factors in order to make a determination of the prominence of suicide prevention in treatment planning for a given individual. A new specifier to indicate the presence of mixed symptoms has been added across both the bipolar and the depressive disorders, allowing for the possibility of manic features in individuals with a diagnosis of unipolar depression. A substantial body of research conducted over the last two decades points to the importance of anxiety as relevant to prognosis and treatment decision making. The *with anxious distress* specifier gives the clinician an opportunity to rate the severity of anxious distress in all individuals with bipolar or depressive disorders.

DSM-5® Depressive Disorders: ICD-9-CM and ICD-10-CM Codes

Disorder	ICD-9-CM	ICD-10-CM
Disruptive Mood Dysregulation Disorder	296.99	F34.8
Major Depressive Disorder	See table below	
Persistent Depressive Disorder (Dysthymia)	300.4	F34.1
Premenstrual Dysphoric Disorder	625.4	N94.3
Substance/Medication-Induced Depressive Disorder	See table on next page	
Depressive Disorder Due to Another Condition	293.83	
With depressive features		F06.31
With major depressive–like episode		F06.32
With mixed features		F06.34
Other Specified Depressive Disorder	311	F32.8
Unspecified Depressive Disorder	311	F32.9

Major Depressive Disorder

Severity/course specifier	Single episode	Recurrent episode*
Mild ([DSM-5] p. 188)	296.21 (F32.0)	296.31 (F33.0)
Moderate ([DSM-5] p. 188)	296.22 (F32.1)	296.32 (F33.1)
Severe ([DSM-5] p. 188)	296.23 (F32.2)	296.33 (F33.2)
With psychotic features** ([DSM-5] p. 186)	206.24 (F32.3)	296.34 (F33.3)
In partial remission ([DSM-5] p. 188)	296.25 (F32.4)	296.35 (F33.41)
In full remission ([DSM-5] p. 188)	292.26 (F32.5)	296.36 (F33.42)
Unspecified	296.20 (F32.9)	296.30 (F33.9)

*For an episode to be considered recurrent, there must be an interval of at least 2 consecutive months between separate episodes in which criteria are not met for a major depressive episode. The definitions of specifiers are found on the indicated pages.

**If psychotic features are present, code the "with psychotic features" specifier irrespective of episode severity.

Substance/Medication-Induced Depressive Disorder

	ICD-9-CM	ICD-10-CM		
		With use disorder, mild	With use disorder, moderate or severe	Without use disorder
Alcohol	291.89	F10.14	F10.24	F10.94
Phencyclidine	292.84	F16.14	F16.24	F16.94
Other hallucinogen	292.84	F16.14	F16.24	F16.94
Inhalant	292.84	F18.14	F18.24	F18.94
Opioid	292.84	F11.14	F11.24	F11.94
Sedative, hypnotic, or anxiolytic	292.84	F13.14	F13.24	F13.94
Amphetamine (or other stimulant)	292.84	F15.14	F15.24	F15.94
Cocaine	292.84	F14.14	F14.24	F14.94
Other (or unknown) substance	292.84	F19.14	F19.24	F19.94

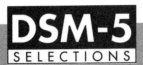

Depressive Disorders

Diagnostic and Statistical Manual of Mental Disorders, Fifth Edition

Depressive disorders include disruptive mood dysregulation disorder, major depressive disorder (including major depressive episode), persistent depressive disorder (dysthymia), premenstrual dysphoric disorder, substance/medication-induced depressive disorder, depressive disorder due to another medical condition, other specified depressive disorder, and unspecified depressive disorder. Unlike in DSM-IV, this chapter "Depressive Disorders" has been separated from the previous chapter "Bipolar and Related Disorders." The common feature of all of these disorders is the presence of sad, empty, or irritable mood, accompanied by somatic and cognitive changes that significantly affect the individual's capacity to function. What differs among them are issues of duration, timing, or presumed etiology.

In order to address concerns about the potential for the overdiagnosis of and treatment for bipolar disorder in children, a new diagnosis, disruptive mood dysregulation disorder, referring to the presentation of children with persistent irritability and frequent episodes of extreme behavioral dyscontrol, is added to the depressive disorders for children up to 12 years of age. Its placement in this chapter reflects the finding that children with this symptom pattern typically develop unipolar depressive disorders or anxiety disorders, rather than bipolar disorders, as they mature into adolescence and adulthood.

Major depressive disorder represents the classic condition in this group of disorders. It is characterized by discrete episodes of at least 2 weeks' duration (although most episodes last considerably longer) involving clear-cut changes in affect, cognition, and neurovegetative functions and inter-episode remissions. A diagnosis based on a single episode is possible, although the disorder is a recurrent one in the majority of cases. Careful consideration is given to the delineation of normal sadness and grief from a major depressive episode. Bereavement may induce great suffering, but it does not typically induce an episode of major depressive disorder. When they do occur together, the depressive symptoms and functional impairment tend to be more severe and the prognosis is worse compared with bereavement that is not accompanied by major depressive disorder. Bereavement-related depression tends to occur in persons with other vulnerabilities to depressive disorders, and recovery may be facilitated by antidepressant treatment.

A more chronic form of depression, persistent depressive disorder (dysthymia), can be diagnosed when the mood disturbance continues for at least 2 years in adults or 1 year in children. This diagnosis, new in DSM-5, includes both the DSM-IV diagnostic categories of chronic major depression and dysthymia.

After careful scientific review of the evidence, premenstrual dysphoric disorder has been moved from an appendix of DSM-IV ("Criteria Sets and Axes Provided for Further Study") to Section II of DSM-5. Almost 20 years of additional research on this condition has confirmed a specific and treatment-responsive form of depressive disorder that begins sometime following ovulation and remits within a few days of menses and has a marked impact on functioning.

A large number of substances of abuse, some prescribed medications, and several medical conditions can be associated with depression-like phenomena. This fact is recognized in the diagnoses of substance/medication-induced depressive disorder and depressive disorder due to another medical condition.

Disruptive Mood Dysregulation Disorder

Diagnostic Criteria	296.99 (F34.8)

A. Severe recurrent temper outbursts manifested verbally (e.g., verbal rages) and/or behaviorally (e.g., physical aggression toward people or property) that are grossly out of proportion in intensity or duration to the situation or provocation.

B. The temper outbursts are inconsistent with developmental level.

C. The temper outbursts occur, on average, three or more times per week.

D. The mood between temper outbursts is persistently irritable or angry most of the day, nearly every day, and is observable by others (e.g., parents, teachers, peers).

E. Criteria A–D have been present for 12 or more months. Throughout that time, the individual has not had a period lasting 3 or more consecutive months without all of the symptoms in Criteria A–D.

F. Criteria A and D are present in at least two of three settings (i.e., at home, at school, with peers) and are severe in at least one of these.

G. The diagnosis should not be made for the first time before age 6 years or after age 18 years.

H. By history or observation, the age at onset of Criteria A–E is before 10 years.

I. There has never been a distinct period lasting more than 1 day during which the full symptom criteria, except duration, for a manic or hypomanic episode have been met.
   Note: Developmentally appropriate mood elevation, such as occurs in the context of a highly positive event or its anticipation, should not be considered as a symptom of mania or hypomania.

J. The behaviors do not occur exclusively during an episode of major depressive disorder and are not better explained by another mental disorder (e.g., autism spectrum disorder, posttraumatic stress disorder, separation anxiety disorder, persistent depressive disorder [dysthymia]).
   Note: This diagnosis cannot coexist with oppositional defiant disorder, intermittent explosive disorder, or bipolar disorder, though it can coexist with others, including major depressive disorder, attention-deficit/hyperactivity disorder, conduct disorder, and substance use disorders. Individuals whose symptoms meet criteria for both disruptive mood dysregulation disorder and oppositional defiant disorder should only be given the diagnosis of disruptive mood dysregulation disorder. If an individual has ever experienced a manic or hypomanic episode, the diagnosis of disruptive mood dysregulation disorder should not be assigned.

K. The symptoms are not attributable to the physiological effects of a substance or to another medical or neurological condition.

Diagnostic Features

The core feature of disruptive mood dysregulation disorder is chronic, severe persistent irritability. This severe irritability has two prominent clinical manifestations, the first of which is frequent temper outbursts. These outbursts typically occur in response to frustration and can be verbal or behavioral (the latter in the form of aggression against property, self, or others). They must occur frequently (i.e., on average, three or more times per week) (Criterion C) over at least 1 year in at least two settings (Criteria E and F), such as in the home and at school, and they must be developmentally inappropriate (Criterion B). The second manifestation of severe irritability consists of chronic, persistently irritable or angry mood that is present between the severe temper outbursts. This irritable or angry mood must be characteristic of the child, being present most of the day, nearly every day, and noticeable by others in the child's environment (Criterion D).

The clinical presentation of disruptive mood dysregulation disorder must be carefully distinguished from presentations of other, related conditions, particularly pediatric bipolar disorder. In fact, disruptive mood dysregulation disorder was added to DSM-5 to address the considerable concern about the appropriate classification and treatment of children who present with chronic, persistent irritability relative to children who present with classic (i.e., episodic) bipolar disorder.

Some researchers view severe, non-episodic irritability as characteristic of bipolar disorder in children, although both DSM-IV and DSM-5 require that both children and adults have distinct episodes of mania or hypomania to qualify for the diagnosis of bipolar I disorder. During the latter decades of the 20th century, this contention by researchers that severe, nonepisodic irritability is a manifestation of pediatric mania coincided with an upsurge in the rates at which clinicians assigned the diagnosis of bipolar disorder to their pediatric patients. This sharp increase in rates appears to be attributable to clinicians combining at least two clinical presentations into a single category. That is, both classic, episodic presentations of mania and non-episodic presentations of severe irritability have been labeled as bipolar disorder in children. In DSM-5, the term *bipolar disorder* is explicitly reserved for episodic presentations of bipolar symptoms. DSM-IV did not include a diagnosis designed to capture youths whose hallmark symptoms consisted of very severe, non-episodic irritability, whereas DSM-5, with the inclusion of disruptive mood dysregulation disorder, provides a distinct category for such presentations.

Prevalence

Disruptive mood dysregulation disorder is common among children presenting to pediatric mental health clinics. Prevalence estimates of the disorder in the community are unclear. Based on rates of chronic and severe persistent irritability, which is the core feature of the disorder, the overall 6-month to 1-year period-prevalence of disruptive mood dysregulation disorder among children and adolescents probably falls in the 2%–5% range. However, rates are expected to be higher in males and school-age children than in females and adolescents.

Development and Course

The onset of disruptive mood dysregulation disorder must be before age 10 years, and the diagnosis should not be applied to children with a developmental age of less than 6 years. It is unknown whether the condition presents only in this age-delimited fashion. Because the symptoms of disruptive mood dysregulation disorder are likely to change as children mature, use of the diagnosis should be restricted to age groups similar to those in which validity has been established (7–18 years). Approximately half of children with severe, chronic irritability will have a presentation that continues to meet criteria for the condition 1 year later. Rates of conversion from severe, nonepisodic irritability to bipolar disorder are very low. Instead, children with chronic irritability are at risk to develop unipolar depressive and/or anxiety disorders in adulthood.

Age-related variations also differentiate classic bipolar disorder and disruptive mood dysregulation disorder. Rates of bipolar disorder generally are very low prior to adolescence (<1%), with a steady increase into early adulthood (1%–2% prevalence). Disruptive mood dysregulation disorder is more common than bipolar disorder prior to adolescence, and symptoms of the condition generally become less common as children transition into adulthood.

Risk and Prognostic Factors

Temperamental.   Children with chronic irritability typically exhibit complicated psychiatric histories. In such children, a relatively extensive history of chronic irritability is common, typically manifesting before full criteria for the syndrome are met. Such prediagnostic presentations may have qualified for a diagnosis of oppositional defiant disorder. Many children with disruptive mood dysregulation disorder have symptoms that also meet criteria for attention-deficit/hyperactivity disorder (ADHD) and for an anxiety disorder, with such diagnoses often being present from a relatively early age. For some children, the criteria for major depressive disorder may also be met.

Genetic and physiological.   In terms of familial aggregation and genetics, it has been suggested that children presenting with chronic, non-episodic irritability can be differentiated from children with bipolar disorder in their family-based risk. However, these two groups do not differ in familial rates of anxiety disorders, unipolar depressive disorders, or substance abuse. Compared with children with pediatric bipolar disorder or other mental illnesses, those with disruptive mood dysregulation disorder exhibit both commonalities and differences in information-processing deficits. For example, face-emotion labeling deficits, as well as perturbed decision making and cognitive control, are present in children with bipolar disorder and chronically irritable children, as well as in children with some other psychiatric conditions. There is also evidence for disorder-specific dysfunction, such as during tasks assessing attention deployment in response to emotional stimuli, which has demonstrated unique signs of dysfunction in children with chronic irritability.

Gender-Related Diagnostic Issues

Children presenting to clinics with features of disruptive mood dysregulation disorder are predominantly male. Among community samples, a male preponderance appears to be supported. This difference in prevalence between males and females differentiates disruptive mood dysregulation disorder from bipolar disorder, in which there is an equal gender prevalence.

Suicide Risk

In general, evidence documenting suicidal behavior and aggression, as well as other severe functional consequences, in disruptive mood dysregulation disorder should be noted when evaluating children with chronic irritability.

Functional Consequences of Disruptive Mood Dysregulation Disorder

Chronic, severe irritability, such as is seen in disruptive mood dysregulation disorder, is associated with marked disruption in a child's family and peer relationships, as well as in school performance. Because of their extremely low frustration tolerance, such children generally have difficulty succeeding in school; they are often unable to participate in the activities typically enjoyed by healthy children; their family life is severely disrupted by their outbursts and irritability; and they have trouble initiating or sustaining friendships. Levels of dysfunction in children with bipolar disorder and disruptive mood dysregulation disorder are generally comparable. Both conditions cause severe disruption in the lives of the affected individual and their families. In both disruptive mood dysregulation disorder and pediatric bipolar disorder, dangerous behavior, suicidal ideation or suicide attempts, severe aggression, and psychiatric hospitalization are common.

Differential Diagnosis

Because chronically irritable children and adolescents typically present with complex histories, the diagnosis of disruptive mood dysregulation disorder must be made while considering the presence or absence of multiple other conditions. Despite the need to consider many other syndromes, differentiation of disruptive mood dysregulation disorder from bipolar disorder and oppositional defiant disorder requires particularly careful assessment.

Bipolar disorders. The central feature differentiating disruptive mood dysregulation disorder and bipolar disorders in children involves the longitudinal course of the core symptoms. In children, as in adults, bipolar I disorder and bipolar II disorder manifest as an episodic illness with discrete episodes of mood perturbation that can be differentiated from the child's typical presentation. The mood perturbation that occurs during a manic episode is distinctly different from the child's usual mood. In addition, during a manic episode, the change in mood must be accompanied by the onset, or worsening, of associated cognitive, behavioral, and physical symptoms (e.g., distractibility, increased goal-directed activity), which are also present to a degree that is distinctly different from the child's usual baseline. Thus, in the case of a manic episode, parents (and, depending on developmental level, children) should be able to identify a distinct time period during which the child's mood and behavior were markedly different from usual. In contrast, the irritability of disruptive mood dysregulation disorder is persistent and is present over many months; while it may wax and wane to a certain degree, severe irritability is characteristic of the child with disruptive mood dysregulation disorder. Thus, while bipolar disorders are episodic conditions, disruptive mood dysregulation disorder is not. In fact, the diagnosis of disruptive mood dysregulation disorder cannot be assigned to a child who has ever experienced a full-duration hypomanic or manic episode (irritable or euphoric) or who has ever had a manic or hypomanic episode lasting more than 1 day. Another central differentiating feature between bipolar disorders and disruptive mood dysregulation disorder is the presence of elevated or expansive mood and grandiosity. These symptoms are common features of mania but are not characteristic of disruptive mood dysregulation disorder.

Oppositional defiant disorder.   While symptoms of oppositional defiant disorder typically do occur in children with disruptive mood dysregulation disorder, mood symptoms of disruptive mood dysregulation disorder are relatively rare in children with oppositional defiant disorder. The key features that warrant the diagnosis of disruptive mood dysregulation disorder in children whose symptoms also meet criteria for oppositional defiant disorder are the presence of severe and frequently recurrent outbursts and a persistent disruption in mood between outbursts. In addition, the diagnosis of disruptive mood dysregulation disorder requires severe impairment in at least one setting (i.e., home, school, or among peers) and mild to moderate impairment in a second setting. For this reason, while most children whose symptoms meet criteria for disruptive mood dysregulation disorder will also have a presentation that meets criteria for oppositional defiant disorder, the reverse is not the case. That is, in only approximately 15% of individuals with oppositional defiant disorder would criteria for disruptive mood dysregulation disorder be met. Moreover, even for children in whom criteria for both disorders are met, only the diagnosis of disruptive mood dysregulation disorder should be made. Finally, both the prominent mood symptoms in disruptive mood dysregulation disorder and the high risk for depressive and anxiety disorders in follow-up studies justify placement of disruptive mood dysregulation disorder among the depressive disorders in DSM-5. (Oppositional defiant disorder is included in the chapter "Disruptive, Impulse-Control, and Conduct Disorders.") This reflects the more prominent mood component among individuals with disruptive mood dysregulation disorder, as compared with individuals with oppositional defiant disorder. Nevertheless, it also should be noted that disruptive mood dysregulation disorder appears to carry a high risk for behavioral problems as well as mood problems.

Attention-deficit/hyperactivity disorder, major depressive disorder, anxiety disorders, and autism spectrum disorder.   Unlike children diagnosed with bipolar disorder or oppositional defiant disorder, a child whose symptoms meet criteria for disruptive mood dysregulation disorder also can receive a comorbid diagnosis of ADHD, major depressive disorder, and/or anxiety disorder. However, children whose irritability is present only in the context of a major depressive episode or persistent depressive disorder (dysthymia) should receive one of those diagnoses rather than disruptive mood dysregulation disorder. Children with disruptive mood dysregulation disorder may have symptoms that also meet criteria for an anxiety disorder and can receive both diagnoses, but children whose irritability is manifest only in the context of exacerbation of an anxiety disorder should receive the relevant anxiety disorder diagnosis rather than disruptive mood dysregulation disorder. In addition, children with autism spectrum disorders frequently present with temper outbursts when, for example, their routines are disturbed. In that instance, the temper outbursts would be considered secondary to the autism spectrum disorder, and the child should not receive the diagnosis of disruptive mood dysregulation disorder.

Intermittent explosive disorder. Children with symptoms suggestive of intermittent explosive disorder present with instances of severe temper outbursts, much like children with disruptive mood dysregulation disorder. However, unlike disruptive mood dysregulation disorder, intermittent explosive disorder does not require persistent disruption in mood between outbursts. In addition, intermittent explosive disorder requires only 3 months of active symptoms, in contrast to the 12-month requirement for disruptive mood dysregulation disorder. Thus, these two diagnoses should not be made in the same child. For children with outbursts and intercurrent, persistent irritability, only the diagnosis of disruptive mood dysregulation disorder should be made.

Comorbidity

Rates of comorbidity in disruptive mood dysregulation disorder are extremely high. It is rare to find individuals whose symptoms meet criteria for disruptive mood dysregulation disorder alone. Comorbidity between disruptive mood dysregulation disorder and other DSM-defined syndromes appears higher than for many other pediatric mental illnesses; the strongest overlap is with oppositional defiant disorder. Not only is the overall rate of comorbidity high in disruptive mood dysregulation disorder, but also the range of comorbid illnesses appears particularly diverse. These children typically present to the clinic with a wide range of disruptive behavior, mood, anxiety, and even autism spectrum symptoms and diagnoses. However, children with disruptive mood dysregulation disorder should not have symptoms that meet criteria for bipolar disorder, as in that context, only the bipolar disorder diagnosis should be made. If children have symptoms that meet criteria for oppositional defiant disorder or intermittent explosive disorder *and* disruptive mood dysregulation disorder, only the diagnosis of disruptive mood dysregulation disorder should be assigned. Also, as noted earlier, the diagnosis of disruptive mood dysregulation disorder should not be assigned if the symptoms occur only in an anxiety-provoking context, when the routines of a child with autism spectrum disorder or obsessive-compulsive disorder are disturbed, or in the context of a major depressive episode.

Major Depressive Disorder

Diagnostic Criteria

A. Five (or more) of the following symptoms have been present during the same 2-week period and represent a change from previous functioning; at least one of the symptoms is either (1) depressed mood or (2) loss of interest or pleasure.
Note: Do not include symptoms that are clearly attributable to another medical condition.

   1. Depressed mood most of the day, nearly every day, as indicated by either subjective report (e.g., feels sad, empty, hopeless) or observation made by others

(e.g., appears tearful). (**Note:** In children and adolescents, can be irritable mood.)

2. Markedly diminished interest or pleasure in all, or almost all, activities most of the day, nearly every day (as indicated by either subjective account or observation).
3. Significant weight loss when not dieting or weight gain (e.g., a change of more than 5% of body weight in a month), or decrease or increase in appetite nearly every day. (**Note:** In children, consider failure to make expected weight gain.)
4. Insomnia or hypersomnia nearly every day.
5. Psychomotor agitation or retardation nearly every day (observable by others, not merely subjective feelings of restlessness or being slowed down).
6. Fatigue or loss of energy nearly every day.
7. Feelings of worthlessness or excessive or inappropriate guilt (which may be delusional) nearly every day (not merely self-reproach or guilt about being sick).
8. Diminished ability to think or concentrate, or indecisiveness, nearly every day (either by subjective account or as observed by others).
9. Recurrent thoughts of death (not just fear of dying), recurrent suicidal ideation without a specific plan, or a suicide attempt or a specific plan for committing suicide.

B. The symptoms cause clinically significant distress or impairment in social, occupational, or other important areas of functioning.

C. The episode is not attributable to the physiological effects of a substance or to another medical condition.

Note: Criteria A–C represent a major depressive episode.

Note: Responses to a significant loss (e.g., bereavement, financial ruin, losses from a natural disaster, a serious medical illness or disability) may include the feelings of intense sadness, rumination about the loss, insomnia, poor appetite, and weight loss noted in Criterion A, which may resemble a depressive episode. Although such symptoms may be understandable or considered appropriate to the loss, the presence of a major depressive episode in addition to the normal response to a significant loss should also be carefully considered. This decision inevitably requires the exercise of clinical judgment based on the individual's history and the cultural norms for the expression of distress in the context of loss.[1]

---

[1] In distinguishing grief from a major depressive episode (MDE), it is useful to consider that in grief the predominant affect is feelings of emptiness and loss, while in MDE it is persistent depressed mood and the inability to anticipate happiness or pleasure. The dysphoria in grief is likely to decrease in intensity over days to weeks and occurs in waves, the so-called pangs of grief. These waves tend to be associated with thoughts or reminders of the deceased. The depressed mood of MDE is more persistent and not tied to specific thoughts or preoccupations. The pain of grief may be accompanied by positive emotions and humor that are uncharacteristic of the pervasive unhappiness and misery characteristic of MDE. The thought content associated with grief generally features a preoccupation with thoughts and memories of the deceased, rather than the self-critical or pessimistic ruminations seen in MDE. In grief, self-esteem is generally preserved, whereas in MDE feelings of worthlessness and self-loathing are common. If self-derogatory ideation is present in grief, it typically involves perceived failings vis-à-vis the deceased (e.g., not visiting frequently enough, not telling the deceased how much he or she was loved). If a bereaved individual thinks about death and dying, such thoughts are generally focused on the deceased and possibly about "joining" the deceased, whereas in MDE such thoughts are focused on ending one's own life because of feeling worthless, undeserving of life, or unable to cope with the pain of depression.

D. The occurrence of the major depressive episode is not better explained by schizo-affective disorder, schizophrenia, schizophreniform disorder, delusional disorder, or other specified and unspecified schizophrenia spectrum and other psychotic disorders.

E. There has never been a manic episode or a hypomanic episode.

> **Note:** This exclusion does not apply if all of the manic-like or hypomanic-like episodes are substance-induced or are attributable to the physiological effects of another medical condition.

Coding and Recording Procedures

The diagnostic code for major depressive disorder is based on whether this is a single or recurrent episode, current severity, presence of psychotic features, and remission status. Current severity and psychotic features are only indicated if full criteria are currently met for a major depressive episode. Remission specifiers are only indicated if the full criteria are not currently met for a major depressive episode. Codes are as follows:

Severity/course specifier	Single episode	Recurrent episode*
Mild ([DSM-5] p. 188)	296.21 (F32.0)	296.31 (F33.0)
Moderate ([DSM-5] p. 188)	296.22 (F32.1)	296.32 (F33.1)
Severe ([DSM-5] p. 188)	296.23 (F32.2)	296.33 (F33.2)
With psychotic features** ([DSM-5] p. 186)	296.24 (F32.3)	296.34 (F33.3)
In partial remission ([DSM-5] p. 188)	296.25 (F32.4)	296.35 (F33.41)
In full remission ([DSM-5] p. 188)	296.26 (F32.5)	296.36 (F33.42)
Unspecified	296.20 (F32.9)	296.30 (F33.9)

*For an episode to be considered recurrent, there must be an interval of at least 2 consecutive months between separate episodes in which criteria are not met for a major depressive episode. The definitions of specifiers are found on the indicated pages.

**If psychotic features are present, code the "with psychotic features" specifier irrespective of episode severity.

In recording the name of a diagnosis, terms should be listed in the following order: major depressive disorder, single or recurrent episode, severity/psychotic/remission specifiers, followed by as many of the following specifiers without codes that apply to the current episode.

Specify:

    With anxious distress ([DSM-5] p. 184)
    With mixed features ([DSM-5] pp. 184–185)
    With melancholic features ([DSM-5] p. 185)
    With atypical features ([DSM-5] pp. 185–186)
    With mood-congruent psychotic features ([DSM-5] p. 186)
    With mood-incongruent psychotic features ([DSM-5] p. 186)
    With catatonia ([DSM-5] p. 186). **Coding note:** Use additional code 293.89 (F06.1).
    With peripartum onset ([DSM-5] pp. 186–187)
    With seasonal pattern (recurrent episode only) ([DSM-5] pp. 187–188)

Diagnostic Features

The criterion symptoms for major depressive disorder must be present nearly every day to be considered present, with the exception of weight change and suicidal ideation. Depressed mood must be present for most of the day, in addition to being present nearly every day. Often insomnia or fatigue is the presenting complaint, and failure to probe for accompanying depressive symptoms will result in underdiagnosis. Sadness may be denied at first but may be elicited through interview or inferred from facial expression and demeanor. With individuals who focus on a somatic complaint, clinicians should determine whether the distress from that complaint is associated with specific depressive symptoms. Fatigue and sleep disturbance are present in a high proportion of cases; psychomotor disturbances are much less common but are indicative of greater overall severity, as is the presence of delusional or near-delusional guilt.

The essential feature of a major depressive episode is a period of at least 2 weeks during which there is either depressed mood or the loss of interest or pleasure in nearly all activities (Criterion A). In children and adolescents, the mood may be irritable rather than sad. The individual must also experience at least four additional symptoms drawn from a list that includes changes in appetite or weight, sleep, and psychomotor activity; decreased energy; feelings of worthlessness or guilt; difficulty thinking, concentrating, or making decisions; or recurrent thoughts of death or suicidal ideation or suicide plans or attempts. To count toward a major depressive episode, a symptom must either be newly present or must have clearly worsened compared with the person's pre-episode status. The symptoms must persist for most of the day, nearly every day, for at least 2 consecutive weeks. The episode must be accompanied by clinically significant distress or impairment in social, occupational, or other important areas of functioning. For some individuals with milder episodes, functioning may appear to be normal but requires markedly increased effort.

The mood in a major depressive episode is often described by the person as depressed, sad, hopeless, discouraged, or "down in the dumps" (Criterion A1). In some cases, sadness may be denied at first but may subsequently be elicited by interview (e.g., by pointing out that the individual looks as if he or she is about to cry). In some individuals who complain of feeling "blah," having no feelings, or feeling anxious, the presence of a depressed mood can be inferred from the person's facial expression and demeanor. Some individuals emphasize somatic complaints (e.g., bodily aches and pains) rather than reporting feelings of sadness. Many individuals report or exhibit increased irritability (e.g., persistent anger, a tendency to respond to events with angry outbursts or blaming others, an exaggerated sense of frustration over minor matters). In children and adolescents, an irritable or cranky mood may develop rather than a sad or dejected mood. This presentation should be differentiated from a pattern of irritability when frustrated.

Loss of interest or pleasure is nearly always present, at least to some degree. Individuals may report feeling less interested in hobbies, "not caring anymore," or not feeling any enjoyment in activities that were previously considered pleasurable (Criterion A2). Family members often notice social withdrawal or neglect of pleasurable avocations (e.g., a formerly avid golfer no longer plays, a child who used to enjoy soccer finds excuses not to practice). In some individuals, there is a significant reduction from previous levels of sexual interest or desire.

Appetite change may involve either a reduction or increase. Some depressed individuals report that they have to force themselves to eat. Others may eat more and may crave specific foods (e.g., sweets or other carbohydrates). When appetite changes are severe (in either direction), there may be a significant loss or gain in weight, or, in children, a failure to make expected weight gains may be noted (Criterion A3).

Sleep disturbance may take the form of either difficulty sleeping or sleeping excessively (Criterion A4). When insomnia is present, it typically takes the form of middle insomnia (i.e., waking up during the night and then having difficulty returning to sleep) or terminal insomnia (i.e., waking too early and being unable to return to sleep). Initial insomnia (i.e., difficulty falling asleep) may also occur. Individuals who present with oversleeping (hypersomnia) may experience prolonged sleep episodes at night or increased daytime sleep. Sometimes the reason that the individual seeks treatment is for the disturbed sleep.

Psychomotor changes include agitation (e.g., the inability to sit still, pacing, hand-wringing; or pulling or rubbing of the skin, clothing, or other objects) or retardation (e.g., slowed speech, thinking, and body movements; increased pauses before answering; speech that is decreased in volume, inflection, amount, or variety of content, or muteness) (Criterion A5). The psychomotor agitation or retardation must be severe enough to be observable by others and not represent merely subjective feelings.

Decreased energy, tiredness, and fatigue are common (Criterion A6). A person may report sustained fatigue without physical exertion. Even the smallest tasks seem to require substantial effort. The efficiency with which tasks are accomplished may be reduced. For example, an individual may complain that washing and dressing in the morning are exhausting and take twice as long as usual.

The sense of worthlessness or guilt associated with a major depressive episode may include unrealistic negative evaluations of one's worth or guilty preoccupations or ruminations over minor past failings (Criterion A7). Such individuals often misinterpret neutral or trivial day-to-day events as evidence of personal defects and have an exaggerated sense of responsibility for untoward events. The sense of worthlessness or guilt may be of delusional proportions (e.g., an individual who is convinced that he or she is personally responsible for world poverty). Blaming oneself for being sick and for failing to meet occupational or interpersonal responsibilities as a result of the depression is very common and, unless delusional, is not considered sufficient to meet this criterion.

Many individuals report impaired ability to think, concentrate, or make even minor decisions (Criterion A8). They may appear easily distracted or complain of memory difficulties. Those engaged in cognitively demanding pursuits are often unable to function. In children, a precipitous drop in grades may reflect poor concentration. In elderly individuals, memory difficulties may be the chief complaint and may be mistaken for early signs of a dementia ("pseudodementia"). When the major depressive episode is successfully treated, the memory problems often fully abate. However, in some individuals, particularly elderly persons, a major depressive episode may sometimes be the initial presentation of an irreversible dementia.

Thoughts of death, suicidal ideation, or suicide attempts (Criterion A9) are common. They may range from a passive wish not to awaken in the morning or a belief that others would be better off if the individual were dead, to transient but recurrent thoughts of committing suicide, to a specific suicide plan. More severely suicidal individuals may have put their affairs in order (e.g., updated wills, settled debts), acquired needed materials (e.g., a rope or a gun), and chosen a location and time to accomplish the suicide. Motivations for suicide may include a desire to give up in the face of perceived insurmountable obstacles, an intense wish to end what is perceived as an unending and excruciatingly painful emotional state, an inability to foresee any enjoyment in life, or the wish to not be a burden to others. The resolution of such thinking may be a more meaningful measure of diminished suicide risk than denial of further plans for suicide.

The evaluation of the symptoms of a major depressive episode is especially difficult when they occur in an individual who also has a general medical condition (e.g., cancer, stroke, myocardial infarction, diabetes, pregnancy). Some of the criterion signs and symptoms of a major depressive episode are identical to those of general medical conditions (e.g., weight loss with untreated diabetes; fatigue with cancer; hypersomnia early in pregnancy; insomnia later in pregnancy or the postpartum). Such symptoms count toward a major depressive diagnosis except when they are clearly and fully attributable to a general medical condition. Nonvegetative symptoms of dysphoria, anhedonia, guilt or worthlessness, impaired concentration or indecision, and suicidal thoughts should be assessed with particular care in such cases. Definitions of major depressive episodes that have been modified to include only these nonvegetative symptoms appear to identify nearly the same individuals as do the full criteria.

Associated Features Supporting Diagnosis

Major depressive disorder is associated with high mortality, much of which is accounted for by suicide; however, it is not the only cause. For example, depressed individuals admitted to nursing homes have a markedly increased likelihood of death in the first year. Individuals frequently present with tearfulness, irritability, brooding, obsessive rumination, anxiety, phobias, excessive worry over physical health, and complaints of pain (e.g., headaches; joint, abdominal, or other pains). In children, separation anxiety may occur.

Although an extensive literature exists describing neuroanatomical, neuroendocrinological, and neurophysiological correlates of major depressive disorder, no laboratory test has yielded results of sufficient sensitivity and specificity to be used as a diagnostic tool for this disorder. Until recently, hypothalamic-pituitary-adrenal axis hyperactivity had been the most extensively investigated abnormality associated with major depressive episodes, and it appears to be associated with melancholia, psychotic features, and risks for eventual suicide. Molecular studies have also implicated peripheral factors, including genetic variants in neurotrophic factors and pro-inflammatory cytokines. Additionally, functional magnetic resonance imaging studies provide evidence for functional abnormalities in specific neural systems supporting emotion processing, reward seeking, and emotion regulation in adults with major depression.

Prevalence

Twelve-month prevalence of major depressive disorder in the United States is approximately 7%, with marked differences by age group such that the prevalence in 18- to 29-

year-old individuals is threefold higher than the prevalence in individuals age 60 years or older. Females experience 1.5- to 3-fold higher rates than males beginning in early adolescence.

Development and Course

Major depressive disorder may first appear at any age, but the likelihood of onset increases markedly with puberty. In the United States, incidence appears to peak in the 20s; however, first onset in late life is not uncommon.

The course of major depressive disorder is quite variable, such that some individuals rarely, if ever, experience remission (a period of 2 or more months with no symptoms, or only one or two symptoms to no more than a mild degree), while others experience many years with few or no symptoms between discrete episodes. It is important to distinguish individuals who present for treatment during an exacerbation of a chronic depressive illness from those whose symptoms developed recently. Chronicity of depressive symptoms substantially increases the likelihood of underlying personality, anxiety, and substance use disorders and decreases the likelihood that treatment will be followed by full symptom resolution. It is therefore useful to ask individuals presenting with depressive symptoms to identify the last period of at least 2 months during which they were entirely free of depressive symptoms.

Recovery typically begins within 3 months of onset for two in five individuals with major depression and within 1 year for four in five individuals. Recency of onset is a strong determinant of the likelihood of near-term recovery, and many individuals who have been depressed only for several months can be expected to recover spontaneously. Features associated with lower recovery rates, other than current episode duration, include psychotic features, prominent anxiety, personality disorders, and symptom severity.

The risk of recurrence becomes progressively lower over time as the duration of remission increases. The risk is higher in individuals whose preceding episode was severe, in younger individuals, and in individuals who have already experienced multiple episodes. The persistence of even mild depressive symptoms during remission is a powerful predictor of recurrence.

Many bipolar illnesses begin with one or more depressive episodes, and a substantial proportion of individuals who initially appear to have major depressive disorder will prove, in time, to instead have a bipolar disorder. This is more likely in individuals with onset of the illness in adolescence, those with psychotic features, and those with a family history of bipolar illness. The presence of a "with mixed features" specifier also increases the risk for future manic or hypomanic diagnosis. Major depressive disorder, particularly with psychotic features, may also transition into schizophrenia, a change that is much more frequent than the reverse.

Despite consistent differences between genders in prevalence rates for depressive disorders, there appear to be no clear differences by gender in phenomenology, course, or treatment response. Similarly, there are no clear effects of current age on the course or treatment response of major depressive disorder. Some symptom differences exist, though, such that hypersomnia and hyperphagia are more likely in younger individuals, and melancholic symptoms, particularly psychomotor disturbances, are more common in older individuals. The likelihood of suicide attempts lessens in middle and late life, although the risk of completed suicide does not. Depressions with earlier ages at onset are more familial and more likely to involve personality disturbances. The course of major depressive disorder within individuals does not generally change with aging. Mean times to recovery appear to be stable over long periods, and the likelihood of being in an episode does not generally increase or decrease with time.

Risk and Prognostic Factors

Temperamental.   Neuroticism (negative affectivity) is a well-established risk factor for the onset of major depressive disorder, and high levels appear to render individuals more likely to develop depressive episodes in response to stressful life events.

Environmental.   Adverse childhood experiences, particularly when there are multiple experiences of diverse types, constitute a set of potent risk factors for major depressive disorder. Stressful life events are well recognized as precipitants of major depressive episodes, but the presence or absence of adverse life events near the onset of episodes does not appear to provide a useful guide to prognosis or treatment selection.

Genetic and physiological.   First-degree family members of individuals with major depressive disorder have a risk for major depressive disorder two- to fourfold higher than that of the general population. Relative risks appear to be higher for early-onset and recurrent forms. Heritability is approximately 40%, and the personality trait neuroticism accounts for a substantial portion of this genetic liability.

Course modifiers.   Essentially all major nonmood disorders increase the risk of an individual developing depression. Major depressive episodes that develop against the background of another disorder often follow a more refractory course. Substance use, anxiety, and borderline personality disorders are among the most common of these, and the presenting depressive symptoms may obscure and delay their recognition. However, sustained clinical improvement in depressive symptoms may depend on the appropriate treatment of underlying illnesses. Chronic or disabling medical conditions also increase risks for major depressive episodes. Such prevalent illnesses as diabetes, morbid obesity, and cardiovascular disease are often complicated by depressive episodes, and these episodes are more likely to become chronic than are depressive episodes in medically healthy individuals.

Culture-Related Diagnostic Issues

Surveys of major depressive disorder across diverse cultures have shown sevenfold differences in 12-month prevalence rates but much more consistency in female-to-male ratio, mean ages at onset, and the degree to which presence of the disorder raises the likelihood of comorbid substance abuse. While these findings suggest substantial cultural differences in the expression of major depressive disorder, they do not permit simple linkages between particular cultures and the likelihood of specific symptoms. Rather, clinicians should be aware that in most countries the majority of cases of depression go unrecognized in primary care settings and that in many cultures, somatic symptoms are very likely to constitute the presenting complaint. Among the Criterion A symptoms, insomnia and loss of energy are the most uniformly reported.

Gender-Related Diagnostic Issues

Although the most reproducible finding in the epidemiology of major depressive disorder has been a higher prevalence in females, there are no clear differences between genders in symptoms, course, treatment response, or functional consequences. In women, the risk for suicide attempts is higher, and the risk for suicide completion is lower. The disparity in suicide rate by gender is not as great among those with depressive disorders as it is in the population as a whole.

Suicide Risk

The possibility of suicidal behavior exists at all times during major depressive episodes. The most consistently described risk factor is a past history of suicide attempts or threats, but it should be remembered that most completed suicides are not preceded by unsuccessful attempts. Other features associated with an increased risk for completed suicide include male sex, being single or living alone, and having prominent feelings of hopelessness. The presence of borderline personality disorder markedly increases risk for future suicide attempts.

Functional Consequences of Major Depressive Disorder

Many of the functional consequences of major depressive disorder derive from individual symptoms. Impairment can be very mild, such that many of those who interact with the affected individual are unaware of depressive symptoms. Impairment may, however, range to complete incapacity such that the depressed individual is unable to attend to basic self-care needs or is mute or catatonic. Among individuals seen in general medical settings, those with major depressive disorder have more pain and physical illness and greater decreases in physical, social, and role functioning.

Differential Diagnosis

Manic episodes with irritable mood or mixed episodes.   Major depressive episodes with prominent irritable mood may be difficult to distinguish from manic episodes with irritable mood or from mixed episodes. This distinction requires a careful clinical evaluation of the presence of manic symptoms.

Mood disorder due to another medical condition.   A major depressive episode is the appropriate diagnosis if the mood disturbance is not judged, based on individual history, physical examination, and laboratory findings, to be the direct pathophysiological consequence of a specific medical condition (e.g., multiple sclerosis, stroke, hypothyroidism).

Substance/medication-induced depressive or bipolar disorder.   This disorder is distinguished from major depressive disorder by the fact that a substance (e.g., a drug of abuse, a medication, a toxin) appears to be etiologically related to the mood disturbance. For example, depressed mood that occurs only in the context of withdrawal from cocaine would be diagnosed as cocaine-induced depressive disorder.

Attention-deficit/hyperactivity disorder. Distractibility and low frustration tolerance can occur in both ADHD and a major depressive episode; if the criteria are met for both, attention-deficit/hyperactivity disorder may be diagnosed in addition to the mood disorder. However, the clinician must be cautious not to overdiagnose a major depressive episode in children with attention-deficit/hyperactivity disorder whose disturbance in mood is characterized by irritability rather than by sadness or loss of interest.

Adjustment disorder with depressed mood. A major depressive episode that occurs in response to a psychosocial stressor is distinguished from adjustment disorder with depressed mood by the fact that the full criteria for a major depressive episode are not met in adjustment disorder.

Sadness. Finally, periods of sadness are inherent aspects of the human experience. These periods should not be diagnosed as a major depressive episode unless criteria are met for severity (i.e., five out of nine symptoms), duration (i.e., most of the day, nearly every day for at least 2 weeks), and clinically significant distress or impairment. The diagnosis other specified depressive disorder may be appropriate for presentations of depressed mood with clinically significant impairment that do not meet criteria for duration or severity.

Comorbidity

Other disorders with which major depressive disorder frequently co-occurs are substance-related disorders, panic disorder, obsessive-compulsive disorder, anorexia nervosa, bulimia nervosa, and borderline personality disorder.

Persistent Depressive Disorder (Dysthymia)

Diagnostic Criteria   **300.4 (F34.1)**

This disorder represents a consolidation of DSM-IV-defined chronic major depressive disorder and dysthymic disorder.

A. Depressed mood for most of the day, for more days than not, as indicated by either subjective account or observation by others, for at least 2 years.

   Note: In children and adolescents, mood can be irritable and duration must be at least 1 year.

B. Presence, while depressed, of two (or more) of the following:

   1. Poor appetite or overeating.
   2. Insomnia or hypersomnia.
   3. Low energy or fatigue.
   4. Low self-esteem.
   5. Poor concentration or difficulty making decisions.
   6. Feelings of hopelessness.

C. During the 2-year period (1 year for children or adolescents) of the disturbance, the individual has never been without the symptoms in Criteria A and B for more than 2 months at a time.

D. Criteria for a major depressive disorder may be continuously present for 2 years.

E. There has never been a manic episode or a hypomanic episode, and criteria have never been met for cyclothymic disorder.

F. The disturbance is not better explained by a persistent schizoaffective disorder, schizophrenia, delusional disorder, or other specified or unspecified schizophrenia spectrum and other psychotic disorder.

G. The symptoms are not attributable to the physiological effects of a substance (e.g., a drug of abuse, a medication) or another medical condition (e.g. hypothyroidism).

H. The symptoms cause clinically significant distress or impairment in social, occupational, or other important areas of functioning.

Note: Because the criteria for a major depressive episode include four symptoms that are absent from the symptom list for persistent depressive disorder (dysthymia), a very limited number of individuals will have depressive symptoms that have persisted longer than 2 years but will not meet criteria for persistent depressive disorder. If full criteria for a major depressive episode have been met at some point during the current episode of illness, they should be given a diagnosis of major depressive disorder. Otherwise, a diagnosis of other specified depressive disorder or unspecified depressive disorder is warranted.

Specify if:
With anxious distress ([DSM-5] p. 184)
With mixed features ([DSM-5] pp. 184–185)
With melancholic features ([DSM-5] p. 185)
With atypical features ([DSM-5] pp. 185–186)
With mood-congruent psychotic features ([DSM-5] p. 186)
With mood-incongruent psychotic features ([DSM-5] p. 186)
With peripartum onset ([DSM-5] pp. 186–187)

Specify if:
In partial remission ([DSM-5] p. 188)
In full remission ([DSM-5] p. 188)

Specify if:
Early onset: If onset is before age 21 years.
Late onset: If onset is at age 21 years or older.

Specify if (for most recent 2 years of persistent depressive disorder):
With pure dysthymic syndrome: Full criteria for a major depressive episode have not been met in at least the preceding 2 years.
With persistent major depressive episode: Full criteria for a major depressive episode have been met throughout the preceding 2-year period.
With intermittent major depressive episodes, with current episode: Full criteria for a major depressive episode are currently met, but there have been periods of at least 8 weeks in at least the preceding 2 years with symptoms below the threshold for a full major depressive episode.
With intermittent major depressive episodes, without current episode: Full criteria for a major depressive episode are not currently met, but there has been one or more major depressive episodes in at least the preceding 2 years.

Specify current severity:
Mild ([DSM-5] p. 188)
Moderate ([DSM-5] p. 188)
Severe ([DSM-5] p. 188)

Diagnostic Features

The essential feature of persistent depressive disorder (dysthymia) is a depressed mood that occurs for most of the day, for more days than not, for at least 2 years, or at least 1 year for children and adolescents (Criterion A). This disorder represents a consolidation of DSM-IV-defined chronic major depressive disorder and dysthymic disorder. Major depression may precede persistent depressive disorder, and major depressive episodes may occur during persistent depressive disorder. Individuals whose symptoms meet major depressive disorder criteria for 2 years should be given a diagnosis of persistent depressive disorder as well as major depressive disorder.

Individuals with persistent depressive disorder describe their mood as sad or "down in the dumps." During periods of depressed mood, at least two of the six symptoms from Criterion B are present. Because these symptoms have become a part of the individual's day-to-day experience, particularly in the case of early onset (e.g., "I've always been this way"), they may not be reported unless the individual is directly prompted. During the 2-year period (1 year for children or adolescents), any symptom-free intervals last no longer than 2 months (Criterion C).

Prevalence

Persistent depressive disorder is effectively an amalgam of DSM-IV dysthymic disorder and chronic major depressive episode. The 12-month prevalence in the United States is approximately 0.5% for persistent depressive disorder and 1.5% for chronic major depressive disorder.

Development and Course

Persistent depressive disorder often has an early and insidious onset (i.e., in childhood, adolescence, or early adult life) and, by definition, a chronic course. Among individuals with both persistent depressive disorder and borderline personality disorder, the covariance of the corresponding features over time suggests the operation of a common mechanism. Early onset (i.e., before age 21 years) is associated with a higher likelihood of comorbid personality disorders and substance use disorders.

When symptoms rise to the level of a major depressive episode, they are likely to subsequently revert to a lower level. However, depressive symptoms are much less likely to resolve in a given period of time in the context of persistent depressive disorder than they are in a major depressive episode.

Risk and Prognostic Factors

Temperamental.   Factors predictive of poorer long-term outcome include higher levels of neuroticism (negative affectivity), greater symptom severity, poorer global functioning, and presence of anxiety disorders or conduct disorder.

Environmental. Childhood risk factors include parental loss or separation.

Genetic and physiological. There are no clear differences in illness development, course, or family history between DSM-IV dysthymic disorder and chronic major depressive disorder. Earlier findings pertaining to either disorder are therefore likely to apply to persistent depressive disorder. It is thus likely that individuals with persistent depressive disorder will have a higher proportion of first-degree relatives with persistent depressive disorder than do individuals with major depressive disorder, and more depressive disorders in general.

A number of brain regions (e.g., prefrontal cortex, anterior cingulate, amygdala, hippocampus) have been implicated in persistent depressive disorder. Possible polysomnographic abnormalities exist as well.

Functional Consequences of Persistent Depressive Disorder

The degree to which persistent depressive disorder impacts social and occupational functioning is likely to vary widely, but effects can be as great as or greater than those of major depressive disorder.

Differential Diagnosis

Major depressive disorder. If there is a depressed mood plus two or more symptoms meeting criteria for a persistent depressive episode for 2 years or more, then the diagnosis of persistent depressive disorder is made. The diagnosis depends on the 2-year duration, which distinguishes it from episodes of depression that do not last 2 years. If the symptom criteria are sufficient for a diagnosis of a major depressive episode at any time during this period, then the diagnosis of major depression should be noted, but it is coded not as a separate diagnosis but rather as a specifier with the diagnosis of persistent depressive disorder. If the individual's symptoms currently meet full criteria for a major depressive episode, then the specifier of "with intermittent major depressive episodes, with current episode" would be made. If the major depressive episode has persisted for at least a 2-year duration and remains present, then the specifier "with persistent major depressive episode" is used. When full major depressive episode criteria are not currently met but there has been at least one previous episode of major depression in the context of at least 2 years of persistent depressive symptoms, then the specifier of "with intermittent major depressive episodes, without current episode" is used. If the individual has not experienced an episode of major depression in the last 2 years, then the specifier "with pure dysthymic syndrome" is used.

Psychotic disorders. Depressive symptoms are a common associated feature of chronic psychotic disorders (e.g., schizoaffective disorder, schizophrenia, delusional disorder). A separate diagnosis of persistent depressive disorder is not made if the symptoms occur only during the course of the psychotic disorder (including residual phases).

Depressive or bipolar and related disorder due to another medical condition. Persistent depressive disorder must be distinguished from a depressive or bipolar and related disorder due to another medical condition. The diagnosis is depressive or bipolar and related disorder due to another medical condition if the mood disturbance is judged, based on history, physical examination, or laboratory findings, to be attributable to the direct pathophysiological effects of a specific, usually chronic, medical condition (e.g., multiple sclerosis). If it is judged that the depressive symptoms are not attributable to the physiological effects of another medical condition, then the primary mental disorder (e.g., persistent depressive disorder) is recorded, and the medical condition is noted as a concomitant medical condition (e.g., diabetes mellitus).

Substance/medication-induced depressive or bipolar disorder. A substance/medication-induced depressive or bipolar and related disorder is distinguished from persistent depressive disorder when a substance (e.g., a drug of abuse, a medication, a toxin) is judged to be etiologically related to the mood disturbance.

Personality disorders. Often, there is evidence of a coexisting personality disturbance. When an individual's presentation meets the criteria for both persistent depressive disorder and a personality disorder, both diagnoses are given.

Comorbidity

In comparison to individuals with major depressive disorder, those with persistent depressive disorder are at higher risk for psychiatric comorbidity in general, and for anxiety disorders and substance use disorders in particular. Early-onset persistent depressive disorder is strongly associated with DSM-IV Cluster B and C personality disorders.

Premenstrual Dysphoric Disorder

Diagnostic Criteria   **625.4 (N94.3)**

A. In the majority of menstrual cycles, at least five symptoms must be present in the final week before the onset of menses, start to *improve* within a few days after the onset of menses, and become *minimal* or absent in the week postmenses.

B. One (or more) of the following symptoms must be present:
1. Marked affective lability (e.g., mood swings; feeling suddenly sad or tearful, or increased sensitivity to rejection).
2. Marked irritability or anger or increased interpersonal conflicts.
3. Marked depressed mood, feelings of hopelessness, or self-deprecating thoughts.
4. Marked anxiety, tension, and/or feelings of being keyed up or on edge.

C. One (or more) of the following symptoms must additionally be present, to reach a total of *five* symptoms when combined with symptoms from Criterion B above.
1. Decreased interest in usual activities (e.g., work, school, friends, hobbies).
2. Subjective difficulty in concentration.
3. Lethargy, easy fatigability, or marked lack of energy.
4. Marked change in appetite; overeating; or specific food cravings.
5. Hypersomnia or insomnia.

6. A sense of being overwhelmed or out of control.
7. Physical symptoms such as breast tenderness or swelling, joint or muscle pain, a sensation of "bloating," or weight gain.

Note: The symptoms in Criteria A–C must have been met for most menstrual cycles that occurred in the preceding year.

D. The symptoms are associated with clinically significant distress or interference with work, school, usual social activities, or relationships with others (e.g., avoidance of social activities; decreased productivity and efficiency at work, school, or home).

E. The disturbance is not merely an exacerbation of the symptoms of another disorder, such as major depressive disorder, panic disorder, persistent depressive disorder (dysthymia), or a personality disorder (although it may co-occur with any of these disorders).

F. Criterion A should be confirmed by prospective daily ratings during at least two symptomatic cycles. (**Note:** The diagnosis may be made provisionally prior to this confirmation.)

G. The symptoms are not attributable to the physiological effects of a substance (e.g., a drug of abuse, a medication, other treatment) or another medical condition (e.g., hyperthyroidism).

Recording Procedures

If symptoms have not been confirmed by prospective daily ratings of at least two symptomatic cycles, "provisional" should be noted after the name of the diagnosis (i.e., "premenstrual dysphoric disorder, provisional").

Diagnostic Features

The essential features of premenstrual dysphoric disorder are the expression of mood lability, irritability, dysphoria, and anxiety symptoms that occur repeatedly during the premenstrual phase of the cycle and remit around the onset of menses or shortly thereafter. These symptoms may be accompanied by behavioral and physical symptoms. Symptoms must have occurred in most of the menstrual cycles during the past year and must have an adverse effect on work or social functioning. The intensity and/or expressivity of the accompanying symptoms may be closely related to social and cultural background characteristics of the affected female, family perspectives, and more specific factors such as religious beliefs, social tolerance, and female gender role issues.

Typically, symptoms peak around the time of the onset of menses. Although it is not uncommon for symptoms to linger into the first few days of menses, the individual must have a symptom-free period in the follicular phase after the menstrual period begins. While the core symptoms include mood and anxiety symptoms, behavioral and somatic symptoms commonly also occur. However, the presence of physical and/or behavioral symptoms in the absence of mood and/or anxious symptoms is not sufficient for a diagnosis. Symptoms are of comparable severity (but not duration) to those of another mental disorder, such as a major depressive episode or generalized anxiety disorder. In order to confirm a provisional diagnosis, daily prospective symptom ratings are required for at least two symptomatic cycles.

Associated Features Supporting Diagnosis

Delusions and hallucinations have been described in the late luteal phase of the menstrual cycle but are rare. The premenstrual phase has been considered by some to be a risk period for suicide.

Prevalence

Twelve-month prevalence of premenstrual dysphoric disorder is between 1.8% and 5.8% of menstruating women. Estimates are substantially inflated if they are based on retrospective reports rather than prospective daily ratings. However, estimated prevalence based on a daily record of symptoms for 1–2 months may be less representative, as individuals with the most severe symptoms may be unable to sustain the rating process. The most rigorous estimate of premenstrual dysphoric disorder is 1.8% for women whose symptoms meet the full criteria without functional impairment and 1.3% for women whose symptoms meet the current criteria with functional impairment and without co-occurring symptoms from another mental disorder.

Development and Course

Onset of premenstrual dysphoric disorder can occur at any point after menarche. Incidence of new cases over a 40-month follow-up period is 2.5% (95% confidence interval [CI] = 1.7–3.7). Anecdotally, many individuals, as they approach menopause, report that symptoms worsen. Symptoms cease after menopause, although cyclical hormone replacement can trigger the re-expression of symptoms.

Risk and Prognostic Factors

Environmental. Environmental factors associated with the expression of premenstrual dysphoric disorder include stress, history of interpersonal trauma, seasonal changes, and sociocultural aspects of female sexual behavior in general, and female gender role in particular.

Genetic and physiological. Heritability of premenstrual dysphoric disorder is unknown. However, for premenstrual symptoms, estimates for heritability range between 30% and 80%, with the most stable component of premenstrual symptoms estimated to be about 50% heritable.

Course modifiers. Women who use oral contraceptives may have fewer premenstrual complaints than do women who do not use oral contraceptives.

Culture-Related Diagnostic Issues

Premenstrual dysphoric disorder is not a culture-bound syndrome and has been observed in individuals in the United States, Europe, India, and Asia. It is unclear as to whether rates differ by race. Nevertheless, frequency, intensity, and expressivity of symptoms and help-seeking patterns may be significantly influenced by cultural factors.

Diagnostic Markers

As indicated earlier, the diagnosis of premenstrual dysphoric disorder is appropriately confirmed by 2 months of prospective symptom ratings. A number of scales, including the Daily Rating of Severity of Problems and the Visual Analogue Scales for Premenstrual Mood Symptoms, have undergone validation and are commonly used in clinical trials for premenstrual dysphoric disorder. The Premenstrual Tension Syndrome Rating Scale has a self-report and an observer version, both of which have been validated and used widely to measure illness severity in women who have premenstrual dysphoric disorder.

Functional Consequences of Premenstrual Dysphoric Disorder

Symptoms must be associated with clinically meaningful distress and/or an obvious and marked impairment in the ability to function socially or occupationally in the week prior to menses. Impairment in social functioning may be manifested by marital discord and problems with children, other family members, or friends. Chronic marital or job problems should not be confused with dysfunction that occurs only in association with premenstrual dysphoric disorder.

Differential Diagnosis

Premenstrual syndrome.   Premenstrual syndrome differs from premenstrual dysphoric disorder in that a minimum of five symptoms is not required, and there is no stipulation of affective symptoms for individuals who have premenstrual syndrome. This condition may be more common than premenstrual dysphoric disorder, although the estimated prevalence of premenstrual syndrome varies. While premenstrual syndrome shares the feature of symptom expression during the premenstrual phase of the menstrual cycle, it is generally considered to be less severe than premenstrual dysphoric disorder. The presence of physical or behavioral symptoms in the premenstruum, without the required affective symptoms, likely meets criteria for premenstrual syndrome and not for premenstrual dysphoric disorder.

Dysmenorrhea.   Dysmenorrhea is a syndrome of painful menses, but this is distinct from a syndrome characterized by affective changes. Moreover, symptoms of dysmenorrhea begin with the onset of menses, whereas symptoms of premenstrual dysphoric disorder, by definition, begin before the onset of menses, even if they linger into the first few days of menses.

Bipolar disorder, major depressive disorder, and persistent depressive disorder (dysthymia).   Many women with (either naturally occurring or substance/medication-induced) bipolar or major depressive disorder or persistent depressive disorder believe that they have premenstrual dysphoric disorder. However, when they chart symptoms, they realize that the symptoms do not follow a premenstrual pattern. Women with another mental disorder may experience chronic symptoms or intermittent symptoms that are unrelated to menstrual cycle phase. However, because the onset of menses constitutes a memorable event, they may report that symptoms occur only during the premenstruum or that symptoms worsen premenstrually. This is one of the rationales for the requirement that symptoms be confirmed by daily prospective ratings. The process of differential diagnosis, particularly if the clinician relies on retrospective symptoms only, is made more difficult because of the overlap between symptoms of premenstrual dysphoric disorder and some other diagnoses. The overlap of symptoms is particularly salient for differentiating premenstrual dysphoric disorder from major depressive episodes, persistent depressive disorder, bipolar disorders, and borderline personality disorder. However, the rate of personality disorders is no higher in individuals with premenstrual dysphoric disorder than in those without the disorder.

Use of hormonal treatments.   Some women who present with moderate to severe premenstrual symptoms may be using hormonal treatments, including hormonal contraceptives. If such symptoms occur after initiation of exogenous hormone use, the symptoms may be due to the use of hormones rather than to the underlying condition of premenstrual dysphoric disorder. If the woman stops hormones and the symptoms disappear, this is consistent with substance/medication-induced depressive disorder.

Comorbidity

A major depressive episode is the most frequently reported previous disorder in individuals presenting with premenstrual dysphoric disorder. A wide range of medical (e.g., migraine, asthma, allergies, seizure disorders) or other mental disorders (e.g., depressive and bipolar disorders, anxiety disorders, bulimia nervosa, substance use disorders) may worsen in the premenstrual phase; however, the absence of a symptom-free period during the postmenstrual interval obviates a diagnosis of premenstrual dysphoric disorder. These conditions are better considered premenstrual exacerbation of a current mental or medical disorder. Although the diagnosis of premenstrual dysphoric disorder should not be assigned in situations in which an individual only experiences a premenstrual exacerbation of another mental or physical disorder, it can be considered in addition to the diagnosis of another mental or physical disorder if the individual experiences symptoms and changes in level of functioning that are characteristic of premenstrual dysphoric disorder and markedly different from the symptoms experienced as part of the ongoing disorder.

Substance/Medication-Induced Depressive Disorder

Diagnostic Criteria

A. A prominent and persistent disturbance in mood that predominates in the clinical picture and is characterized by depressed mood or markedly diminished interest or pleasure in all, or almost all, activities.

B. There is evidence from the history, physical examination, or laboratory findings of both (1) and (2):

1. The symptoms in Criterion A developed during or soon after substance intoxication or withdrawal or after exposure to a medication.

2. The involved substance/medication is capable of producing the symptoms in Criterion A.

C. The disturbance is not better explained by a depressive disorder that is not substance/ medication-induced. Such evidence of an independent depressive disorder could include the following:

The symptoms preceded the onset of the substance/medication use; the symptoms persist for a substantial period of time (e.g., about 1 month) after the cessation of acute withdrawal or severe intoxication; or there is other evidence suggesting the existence of an independent non-substance/medication-induced depressive disorder (e.g., a history of recurrent non-substance/medication-related episodes).

D. The disturbance does not occur exclusively during the course of a delirium.

E. The disturbance causes clinically significant distress or impairment in social, occupational, or other important areas of functioning.

Note: This diagnosis should be made instead of a diagnosis of substance intoxication or substance withdrawal only when the symptoms in Criterion A predominate in the clinical picture and when they are sufficiently severe to warrant clinical attention.

Coding note: The ICD-9-CM and ICD-10-CM codes for the [specific substance/ medication]-induced depressive disorders are indicated in the table below. Note that the ICD-10-CM code depends on whether or not there is a comorbid substance use disorder present for the same class of substance. If a mild substance use disorder is comorbid with the substance-induced depressive disorder, the 4th position character is "1," and the clinician should record "mild [substance] use disorder" before the substance-induced depressive disorder (e.g., "mild cocaine use disorder with cocaine-induced depressive disorder"). If a moderate or severe substance use disorder is comorbid with the substance-induced depressive disorder, the 4th position character is "2," and the clinician should record "moderate [substance] use disorder" or "severe [substance] use disorder," depending on the severity of the comorbid substance use disorder. If there is no comorbid substance use disorder (e.g., after a one-time heavy use of the substance), then the 4th position character is "9," and the clinician should record only the substance-induced depressive disorder.

		ICD-10-CM		
	ICD-9-CM	With use disorder, mild	With use disorder, moderate or severe	Without use disorder
Alcohol	291.89	F10.14	F10.24	F10.94
Phencyclidine	292.84	F16.14	F16.24	F16.94
Other hallucinogen	292.84	F16.14	F16.24	F16.94
Inhalant	292.84	F18.14	F18.24	F18.94
Opioid	292.84	F11.14	F11.24	F11.94
Sedative, hypnotic, or anxiolytic	292.84	F13.14	F13.24	F13.94
Amphetamine (or other stimulant)	292.84	F15.14	F15.24	F15.94
Cocaine	292.84	F14.14	F14.24	F14.94
Other (or unknown) substance	292.84	F19.14	F19.24	F19.94

Specify if (see Table 1 in the chapter "Substance-Related and Addictive Disorders" [in DSM-5] for diagnoses associated with substance class):

With onset during intoxication: If criteria are met for intoxication with the substance and the symptoms develop during intoxication.

With onset during withdrawal: If criteria are met for withdrawal from the substance and the symptoms develop during, or shortly after, withdrawal.

Recording Procedures

ICD-9-CM. The name of the substance/medication-induced depressive disorder begins with the specific substance (e.g., cocaine, dexamethasone) that is presumed to be causing the depressive symptoms. The diagnostic code is selected from the table included in the criteria set, which is based on the drug class. For substances that do not fit into any of the classes (e.g., dexamethasone), the code for "other substance" should be used; and in cases in which a substance is judged to be an etiological factor but the specific class of substance is unknown, the category "unknown substance" should be used.

The name of the disorder is followed by the specification of onset (i.e., onset during intoxication, onset during withdrawal). Unlike the recording procedures for ICD-10-CM, which combine the substance-induced disorder and substance use disorder into a single code, for ICD-9-CM a separate diagnostic code is given for the substance use disorder. For example, in the case of depressive symptoms occurring during withdrawal in a man with a severe cocaine use disorder, the diagnosis is 292.84 cocaine-induced depressive disorder, with onset during withdrawal. An additional diagnosis of 304.20 severe cocaine use disorder is also given. When more than one substance is judged to play a significant role in the development of depressive mood symptoms, each should be listed separately (e.g., 292.84 methylphenidate-induced depressive disorder, with onset during withdrawal; 292.84 dexamethasone-induced depressive disorder, with onset during intoxication).

ICD-10-CM. The name of the substance/medication-induced depressive disorder begins with the specific substance (e.g., cocaine, dexamethasone) that is presumed to be causing the depressive symptoms. The diagnostic code is selected from the table included in the criteria set, which is based on the drug class and presence or absence of a comorbid substance use disorder. For substances that do not fit into any of the classes (e.g., dexamethasone), the code for "other substance" should be used; and in cases in which a substance is judged to be an etiological factor but the specific class of substance is unknown, the category "unknown substance" should be used.

When recording the name of the disorder, the comorbid substance use disorder (if any) is listed first, followed by the word "with," followed by the name of the substance-induced depressive disorder, followed by the specification of onset (i.e., onset during intoxication, onset during withdrawal). For example, in the case of depressive symptoms occurring during withdrawal in a man with a severe cocaine use disorder, the diagnosis is F14.24 severe cocaine use disorder with cocaine-induced depressive disorder, with onset during withdrawal. A separate diagnosis of the comorbid severe cocaine use disorder is not given. If the substance-induced depressive disorder occurs without a comorbid substance use disorder (e.g., after a one-time heavy use of the substance), no accompanying substance use disorder is noted (e.g., F16.94 phencyclidine-induced depressive disorder, with onset during intoxication). When more than one substance is judged to play a significant role in the development of depressive mood symptoms, each should be listed separately (e.g., F15.24 severe methylphenidate use disorder with methylphenidate-induced depressive disorder, with onset during withdrawal; F19.94 dexamethasone-induced depressive disorder, with onset during intoxication).

Diagnostic Features

The diagnostic features of substance/medication-induced depressive disorder include the symptoms of a depressive disorder, such as major depressive disorder; however, the depressive symptoms are associated with the ingestion, injection, or inhalation of a substance (e.g., drug of abuse, toxin, psychotropic medication, other medication), and the depressive symptoms persist beyond the expected length of physiological effects, intoxication, or withdrawal period. As evidenced by clinical history, physical examination, or laboratory findings, the relevant depressive disorder should have developed during or within 1 month after use of a substance that is capable of producing the depressive disorder (Criterion B1). In addition, the diagnosis is not better explained by an independent depressive disorder. Evidence of an independent depressive disorder includes the depressive disorder preceded the onset of ingestion or withdrawal from the substance; the depressive disorder persists beyond a substantial period of time after the cessation of substance use; or other evidence suggests the existence of an independent non-substance/medication-induced depressive disorder (Criterion C). This diagnosis should not be made when symptoms occur exclusively during the course of a delirium (Criterion D). The depressive disorder associated with the substance use, intoxication, or withdrawal must cause clinically significant distress or impairment in social, occupational, or other important areas of functioning to qualify for this diagnosis (Criterion E).

Some medications (e.g., stimulants, steroids, L-dopa, antibiotics, central nervous system drugs, dermatological agents, chemotherapeutic drugs, immunological agents) can induce depressive mood disturbances. Clinical judgment is essential to determine whether the medication is truly associated with inducing the depressive disorder or whether a primary depressive disorder happened to have its onset while the person was receiving the treatment. For example, a depressive episode that developed within the first several weeks of beginning alpha-methyldopa (an antihypertensive agent) in an individual with no history of major depressive disorder would qualify for the diagnosis of medication-induced depressive disorder. In some cases, a previously established condition (e.g., major depressive disorder, recurrent) can recur while the individual is coincidentally taking a medication that has the capacity to cause depressive symptoms (e.g., L-dopa, oral contraceptives). In such cases, the clinician must make a judgment as to whether the medication is causative in this particular situation.

A substance/medication-induced depressive disorder is distinguished from a primary depressive disorder by considering the onset, course, and other factors associated with the substance use. There must be evidence from the history, physical examination, or laboratory findings of substance use, abuse, intoxication, or withdrawal prior to the onset of the depressive disorder. The withdrawal state for some substances can be relatively protracted, and thus intense depressive symptoms can last for a long period after the cessation of substance use.

Prevalence

In a nationally representative U.S. adult population, the lifetime prevalence of substance/medication-induced depressive disorder is 0.26%.

Development and Course

A depressive disorder associated with the use of substance (i.e., alcohol, illicit drugs, or a prescribed treatment for a mental disorder or another medical condition) must have its onset while the individual is using the substance or during withdrawal, if there is a withdrawal syndrome associated with the substance. Most often, the depressive disorder has its onset within the first few weeks or 1 month of use of the substance. Once the substance is discontinued, the depressive symptoms usually remit within days to several weeks, depending on the half-life of the substance/medication and the presence of a withdrawal syndrome. If symptoms persist 4 weeks beyond the expected time course of withdrawal of a particular substance/medication, other causes for the depressive mood symptoms should be considered.

Although there are a few prospective controlled trials examining the association of depressive symptoms with use of a medication, most reports are from postmarketing surveillance studies, retrospective observational studies, or case reports, making evidence of causality difficult to determine. Substances implicated in medication-induced depressive disorder, with varying degrees of evidence, include antiviral agents (efavirenz), cardiovascular agents (clonidine, guanethidine, methyldopa, reserpine), retinoic acid derivatives (isotretinoin), antidepressants, anticonvulsants, anti-migraine agents (triptans), antipsychotics, hormonal agents (corticosteroids, oral contraceptives, gonadotropin-releasing hormone agonists, tamoxifen), smoking cessation agents (varenicline), and immunological agents (interferon). However, other potential substances continue to emerge as new compounds are synthesized. A history of such substance use may help increase diagnostic certainty.

Risk and Prognostic Factors

Temperamental.   Factors that appear to increase the risk of substance/medication-induced depressive disorder can be conceptualized as pertaining to the specific type of drug or to a group of individuals with underlying alcohol or drug use disorders. Risk factors common to all drugs include history of major depressive disorder, history of drug-induced depression, and psychosocial stressors.

Environmental.   There are also risks factors pertaining to a specific type of medication (e.g., increased immune activation prior to treatment for hepatitis C associated with interferon-alfa-induced depression); high doses (greater than 80 mg/day prednisone-equivalents) of corticosteroids or high plasma concentrations of efavirenz; and high estrogen/progesterone content in oral contraceptives.

Course modifiers. In a representative U.S. adult population, compared with individuals with major depressive disorder who did not have a substance use disorder, individuals with substance-induced depressive disorder were more likely to be male, to be black, to have at most a high school diploma, to lack insurance, and to have lower family income. They were also more likely to report higher family history of substance use disorders and antisocial behavior, higher 12-month history of stressful life events, and a greater number of DSM-IV major depressive disorder criteria. They were more likely to report feelings of worthlessness, insomnia/hypersomnia, and thoughts of death and suicide attempts, but less likely to report depressed mood and parental loss by death before age 18 years.

Diagnostic Markers

Determination of the substance of use can sometimes be made through laboratory assays of the suspected substance in the blood or urine to corroborate the diagnosis.

Suicide Risk

Drug-induced or treatment-emergent suicidality represents a marked change in thoughts and behavior from the person's baseline, is usually temporally associated with initiation of a substance, and must be distinguished from the underlying primary mental disorders.

In regard to the treatment-emergent suicidality associated with antidepressants, a U.S. Food and Drug Administration (FDA) advisory committee considered meta-analyses of 99,839 participants enrolled in 372 randomized clinical trials of antidepressants in trials for mental disorders. The analyses showed that when the data were pooled across all adult age groups, there was no perceptible increased risk of suicidal behavior or ideation. However, in age-stratified analyses, the risk for patients ages 18–24 years was elevated, albeit not significantly (odds ratio [OR] = 1.55; 95% CI = 0.91–2.70). The FDA meta-analyses reveal an absolute risk of suicide in patients taking investigational antidepressants of 0.01%. In conclusion, suicide is clearly an extremely rare treatment-emergent phenomenon, but the outcome of suicide was serious enough to prompt the FDA to issue an expanded black-box warning in 2007 regarding the importance of careful monitoring of treatment-emergent suicidal ideation in patients receiving antidepressants.

Differential Diagnosis

Substance intoxication and withdrawal. Depressive symptoms occur commonly in substance intoxication and substance withdrawal, and the diagnosis of the substance-specific intoxication or withdrawal will usually suffice to categorize the symptom presentation. A diagnosis of substance-induced depressive disorder should be made instead of a diagnosis of substance intoxication or substance withdrawal when the mood symptoms are sufficiently severe to warrant independent clinical attention. For example, dysphoric mood is a characteristic feature of cocaine withdrawal. Substance/medication-induced depressive disorder should be diagnosed instead of cocaine withdrawal only if the mood disturbance is substantially more intense or longer lasting than what is usually encountered with cocaine withdrawal and is sufficiently severe to be a separate focus of attention and treatment.

Primary depressive disorder. A substance/medication-induced depressive disorder is distinguished from a primary depressive disorder by the fact that a substance is judged to be etiologically related to the symptoms, as described earlier (see section "Development and Course" for this disorder).

Depressive disorder due to another medical condition. Because individuals with other medical conditions often take medications for those conditions, the clinician must consider the possibility that the mood symptoms are caused by the physiological consequences of the medical condition rather than the medication, in which case depressive disorder due to another medical condition is diagnosed. The history often provides the primary basis for such a judgment. At times, a change in the treatment for the other medical condition (e.g., medication substitution or discontinuation) may be needed to determine empirically whether the medication is the causative agent. If the clinician has ascertained that the disturbance is a function of both another medical condition and substance use or withdrawal, both diagnoses (i.e., depressive disorder due to another medical condition and substance/medication-induced depressive disorder) may be given. When there is insufficient evidence to determine whether the depressive symptoms are associated with substance (including a medication) ingestion or withdrawal or with another medical condition or are primary (i.e., not a function of either a substance or another medical condition), a diagnosis of other specified depressive disorder or unspecified depressive disorder would be indicated.

Comorbidity

Compared with individuals with major depressive disorder and no comorbid substance use disorder, those with substance/medication-induced depressive disorder have higher rates of comorbidity with any DSM-IV mental disorder; are more likely to have specific DSM-IV disorders of pathological gambling and paranoid, histrionic, and antisocial personality disorders; and are less likely to have persistent depressive disorder (dysthymia). Compared with individuals with major depressive disorder and a comorbid substance use disorder, individuals with substance/medication-induced depressive disorder are more likely to have alcohol use disorder, any other substance use disorder, and histrionic personality disorder; however, they are less likely to have persistent depressive disorder.

Depressive Disorder Due to Another Medical Condition

Diagnostic Criteria

A. A prominent and persistent period of depressed mood or markedly diminished interest or pleasure in all, or almost all, activities that predominates in the clinical picture.
B. There is evidence from the history, physical examination, or laboratory findings that the disturbance is the direct pathophysiological consequence of another medical condition.
C. The disturbance is not better explained by another mental disorder (e.g., adjustment disorder, with depressed mood, in which the stressor is a serious medical condition).

D. The disturbance does not occur exclusively during the course of a delirium.

E. The disturbance causes clinically significant distress or impairment in social, occupational, or other important areas of functioning.

Coding note: The ICD-9-CM code for depressive disorder due to another medical condition is **293.83,** which is assigned regardless of the specifier. The ICD-10-CM code depends on the specifier (see below).

Specify if:

(F06.31) With depressive features: Full criteria are not met for a major depressive episode.

(F06.32) With major depressive–like episode: Full criteria are met (except Criterion C) for a major depressive episode.

(F06.34) With mixed features: Symptoms of mania or hypomania are also present but do not predominate in the clinical picture.

Coding note: Include the name of the other medical condition in the name of the mental disorder (e.g., 293.83 [F06.31] depressive disorder due to hypothyroidism, with depressive features). The other medical condition should also be coded and listed separately immediately before the depressive disorder due to the medical condition (e.g., 244.9 [E03.9] hypothyroidism; 293.83 [F06.31] depressive disorder due to hypothyroidism, with depressive features).

Diagnostic Features

The essential feature of depressive disorder due to another medical condition is a prominent and persistent period of depressed mood or markedly diminished interest or pleasure in all, or almost all, activities that predominates in the clinical picture (Criterion A) and that is thought to be related to the direct physiological effects of another medical condition (Criterion B). In determining whether the mood disturbance is due to a general medical condition, the clinician must first establish the presence of a general medical condition. Further, the clinician must establish that the mood disturbance is etiologically related to the general medical condition through a physiological mechanism. A careful and comprehensive assessment of multiple factors is necessary to make this judgment. Although there are no infallible guidelines for determining whether the relationship between the mood disturbance and the general medical condition is etiological, several considerations provide some guidance in this area. One consideration is the presence of a temporal association between the onset, exacerbation, or remission of the general medical condition and that of the mood disturbance. A second consideration is the presence of features that are atypical of primary Mood Disorders (e.g., atypical age at onset or course or absence of family history). Evidence from the literature that suggests that there can be a direct association between the general medical condition in question and the development of mood symptoms can provide a useful context in the assessment of a particular situation.

Associated Features Supporting Diagnosis

Etiology (i.e., a causal relationship to another medical condition based on best clinical evidence) is the key variable in depressive disorder due to another medical condition. The listing of the medical conditions that are said to be able to induce major depression is never complete, and the clinician's best judgment is the essence of this diagnosis.

There are clear associations, as well as some neuroanatomical correlates, of depression with stroke, Huntington's disease, Parkinson's disease, and traumatic brain injury. Among the neuroendocrine conditions most closely associated with depression are Cushing's disease and hypothyroidism. There are numerous other conditions thought to be associated with depression, such as multiple sclerosis. However, the literature's support for a causal association is greater with some conditions, such as Parkinson's disease and Huntington's disease, than with others, for which the differential diagnosis may be adjustment disorder, with depressed mood.

Development and Course

Following stroke, the onset of depression appears to be very acute, occurring within 1 day or a few days of the cerebrovascular accident (CVA) in the largest case series. However, in some cases, onset of the depression is weeks to months following the CVA. In the largest series, the duration of the major depressive episode following stroke was 9–11 months on average. Similarly, in Huntington's disease the depressive state comes quite early in the course of the illness. With Parkinson's disease and Huntington's disease, it often precedes the major motor impairments and cognitive impairments associated with each condition. This is more prominently the case for Huntington's disease, in which depression is considered to be the first neuropsychiatric symptom. There is some observational evidence that depression is less common as the dementia of Huntington's disease progresses.

Risk and Prognostic Factors

The risk of acute onset of a major depressive disorder following a CVA (within 1 day to a week of the event) appears to be strongly correlated with lesion location, with greatest risk associated with left frontal strokes and least risk apparently associated with right frontal lesions in those individuals who present within days of the stroke. The association with frontal regions and laterality is not observed in depressive states that occur in the 2–6 months following stroke.

Gender-Related Diagnostic Issues

Gender differences pertain to those associated with the medical condition (e.g., systemic lupus erythematosus is more common in females; stroke is somewhat more common in middle-age males compared with females).

Diagnostic Markers

Diagnostic markers pertain to those associated with the medical condition (e.g., steroid levels in blood or urine to help corroborate the diagnosis of Cushing's disease, which can be associated with manic or depressive syndromes).

Suicide Risk

There are no epidemiological studies that provide evidence to differentiate the risk of suicide from a major depressive episode due to another medical condition compared with the risk from a major depressive episode in general. There are case reports of suicides in association with major depressive episodes associated with another medical condition. There is a clear association between serious medical illnesses and suicide, particularly shortly after onset or diagnosis of the illness. Thus, it would be prudent to assume that the risk of suicide for major depressive episodes associated with medical conditions is not less than that for other forms of major depressive episode, and might even be greater.

Functional Consequences of Depressive Disorder Due to Another Medical Condition

Functional consequences pertain to those associated with the medical condition. In general, it is believed, but not established, that a major depressive episode induced by Cushing's disease will not recur if the Cushing's disease is cured or arrested. However, it is also suggested, but not established, that mood syndromes, including depressive and manic/hypomanic ones, may be episodic (i.e., recurring) in some individuals with static brain injuries and other central nervous system diseases.

Differential Diagnosis

Depressive disorders not due to another medical condition.   Determination of whether a medical condition accompanying a depressive disorder is causing the disorder depends on a) the absence of an episode(s) of depressive episodes prior to the onset of the medical condition, b) the probability that the associated medical condition has a potential to promote or cause a depressive disorder, and c) a course of the depressive symptoms shortly after the onset or worsening of the medical condition, especially if the depressive symptoms remit near the time that the medical disorder is effectively treated or remits.

Medication-induced depressive disorder.   An important caveat is that some medical conditions are treated with medications (e.g., steroids or alpha-interferon) that can induce depressive or manic symptoms. In these cases, clinical judgment, based on all the evidence in hand, is the best way to try to separate the most likely and/or the most important of two etiological factors (i.e., association with the medical condition vs. a substance-induced syndrome).

Adjustment disorders.   It is important to differentiate a depressive episode from an adjustment disorder, as the onset of the medical condition is in itself a life stressor that could bring on either an adjustment disorder or an episode of major depression. The major differentiating elements are the pervasiveness the depressive picture and the number and quality of the depressive symptoms that the patient reports or demonstrates on the mental status examination. The differential diagnosis of the associated medical conditions is relevant but largely beyond the scope of the present manual.

Comorbidity

Conditions comorbid with depressive disorder due to another medical condition are those associated with the medical conditions of etiological relevance. It has been noted that delirium can occur before or along with depressive symptoms in individuals with a variety of medical conditions, such as Cushing's disease. The association of anxiety symptoms, usually generalized symptoms, is common in depressive disorders, regardless of cause.

Other Specified Depressive Disorder

311 (F32.8)

This category applies to presentations in which symptoms characteristic of a depressive disorder that cause clinically significant distress or impairment in social, occupational, or other important areas of functioning predominate but do not meet the full criteria for any of the disorders in the depressive disorders diagnostic class. The other specified depressive disorder category is used in situations in which the clinician chooses to communicate the specific reason that the presentation does not meet the criteria for any specific depressive disorder. This is done by recording "other specified depressive disorder" followed by the specific reason (e.g., "short-duration depressive episode").

Examples of presentations that can be specified using the "other specified" designation include the following:

1. **Recurrent brief depression:** Concurrent presence of depressed mood and at least four other symptoms of depression for 2–13 days at least once per month (not associated with the menstrual cycle) for at least 12 consecutive months in an individual whose presentation has never met criteria for any other depressive or bipolar disorder and does not currently meet active or residual criteria for any psychotic disorder.

2. **Short-duration depressive episode (4–13 days):** Depressed affect and at least four of the other eight symptoms of a major depressive episode associated with clinically significant distress or impairment that persists for more than 4 days, but less than 14 days, in an individual whose presentation has never met criteria for any other depressive or bipolar disorder, does not currently meet active or residual criteria for any psychotic disorder, and does not meet criteria for recurrent brief depression.

3. **Depressive episode with insufficient symptoms:** Depressed affect and at least one of the other eight symptoms of a major depressive episode associated with clinically significant distress or impairment that persist for at least 2 weeks in an individual whose presentation has never met criteria for any other depressive or bipolar disorder, does not currently meet active or residual criteria for any psychotic disorder, and does not meet criteria for mixed anxiety and depressive disorder symptoms.

Unspecified Depressive Disorder

311 (F32.9)

This category applies to presentations in which symptoms characteristic of a depressive disorder that cause clinically significant distress or impairment in social, occupational, or other important areas of functioning predominate but do not meet the full criteria for any of the disorders in the depressive disorders diagnostic class. The unspecified depressive disorder category is used in situations in which the clinician chooses *not* to specify the reason that the criteria are not met for a specific depressive disorder, and includes presentations for which there is insufficient information to make a more specific diagnosis (e.g., in emergency room settings).

Specifiers for Depressive Disorders

Specify if:

With anxious distress: Anxious distress is defined as the presence of at least two of the following symptoms during the majority of days of a major depressive episode or persistent depressive disorder (dysthymia):

1. Feeling keyed up or tense.
2. Feeling unusually restless.
3. Difficulty concentrating because of worry.
4. Fear that something awful may happen.
5. Feeling that the individual might lose control of himself or herself.

Specify current severity:

Mild: Two symptoms.
Moderate: Three symptoms.
Moderate-severe: Four or five symptoms.
Severe: Four or five symptoms and with motor agitation.

Note: Anxious distress has been noted as a prominent feature of both bipolar and major depressive disorder in both primary care and specialty mental health settings. High levels of anxiety have been associated with higher suicide risk, longer duration of illness, and greater likelihood of treatment nonresponse. As a result, it is clinically useful to specify accurately the presence and severity levels of anxious distress for treatment planning and monitoring of response to treatment.

With mixed features:

A. At least three of the following manic/hypomanic symptoms are present nearly every day during the majority of days of a major depressive episode:

1. Elevated, expansive mood.
2. Inflated self-esteem or grandiosity.
3. More talkative than usual or pressure to keep talking.
4. Flight of ideas or subjective experience that thoughts are racing.
5. Increase in energy or goal-directed activity (either socially, at work or school, or sexually).
6. Increased or excessive involvement in activities that have a high potential for painful consequences (e.g., engaging in unrestrained buying sprees, sexual indiscretions, foolish business investments).
7. Decreased need for sleep (feeling rested despite sleeping less than usual; to be contrasted with insomnia).

B. Mixed symptoms are observable by others and represent a change from the person's usual behavior.

C. For individuals whose symptoms meet full criteria for either mania or hypomania, the diagnosis should be bipolar I or bipolar II disorder.

D. The mixed symptoms are not attributable to the physiological effects of a substance (e.g., a drug of abuse, a medication or other treatment).

Note: Mixed features associated with a major depressive episode have been found to be a significant risk factor for the development of bipolar I or bipolar II disorder. As a result, it is clinically useful to note the presence of this specifier for treatment planning and monitoring of response to treatment.

With melancholic features:

A. One of the following is present during the most severe period of the current episode:

1. Loss of pleasure in all, or almost all, activities.
2. Lack of reactivity to usually pleasurable stimuli (does not feel much better, even temporarily, when something good happens).

B. Three (or more) of the following:

1. A distinct quality of depressed mood characterized by profound despondency, despair, and/or moroseness or by so-called empty mood.
2. Depression that is regularly worse in the morning.
3. Early-morning awakening (i.e., at least 2 hours before usual awakening).
4. Marked psychomotor agitation or retardation.
5. Significant anorexia or weight loss.
6. Excessive or inappropriate guilt.

Note: The specifier "with melancholic features" is applied if these features are present at the most severe stage of the episode. There is a near-complete absence of the capacity for pleasure, not merely a diminution. A guideline for evaluating the lack of reactivity of mood is that even highly desired events are not associated with marked brightening of mood. Either mood does not brighten at all, or it brightens only partially (e.g., up to 20%–40% of normal for only minutes at a time). The "distinct quality" of mood that is characteristic of the "with melancholic features" specifier is experienced as qualitatively different from that during a nonmelancholic depressive episode. A depressed mood that is described as merely more severe, longer lasting, or present without a reason is not considered distinct in quality. Psychomotor changes are nearly always present and are observable by others.

Melancholic features exhibit only a modest tendency to repeat across episodes in the same individual. They are more frequent in inpatients, as opposed to outpatients; are less likely to occur in milder than in more severe major depressive episodes; and are more likely to occur in those with psychotic features.

With atypical features: This specifier can be applied when these features predominate during the majority of days of the current or most recent major depressive episode or persistent depressive disorder.

A. Mood reactivity (i.e., mood brightens in response to actual or potential positive events).

B. Two (or more) of the following:

1. Significant weight gain or increase in appetite.
2. Hypersomnia.
3. Leaden paralysis (i.e., heavy, leaden feelings in arms or legs).
4. A long-standing pattern of interpersonal rejection sensitivity (not limited to episodes of mood disturbance) that results in significant social or occupational impairment.

C. Criteria are not met for "with melancholic features" or "with catatonia" during the same episode.

Note: "Atypical depression" has historical significance (i.e., atypical in contradistinction to the more classical agitated, "endogenous" presentations of depression that were the norm when depression was rarely diagnosed in outpatients and almost never in adolescents or younger adults) and today does not connote an uncommon or unusual clinical presentation as the term might imply.

Mood reactivity is the capacity to be cheered up when presented with positive events (e.g., a visit from children, compliments from others). Mood may become euthymic (not sad) even for extended periods of time if the external circumstances remain favorable. Increased appetite may be manifested by an obvious increase in food intake or by weight gain. Hypersomnia may include either an extended period of nighttime sleep or daytime napping that totals at least 10 hours of sleep per day (or at least 2 hours more than when not depressed). Leaden paralysis is defined as feeling heavy, leaden, or weighted down, usually in the arms or legs. This sensation is generally present for at least an hour a day but often lasts for many hours at a time. Unlike the other atypical features, pathological sensitivity to perceived interpersonal rejection is a trait that has an early onset and persists throughout most of adult life. Rejection sensitivity occurs both when the person is and is not depressed, though it may be exacerbated during depressive periods.

With psychotic features: Delusions and/or hallucinations are present.

> **With mood-congruent psychotic features:** The content of all delusions and hallucinations is consistent with the typical depressive themes of personal inadequacy, guilt, disease, death, nihilism, or deserved punishment.

> **With mood-incongruent psychotic features:** The content of the delusions or hallucinations does not involve typical depressive themes of personal inadequacy, guilt, disease, death, nihilism, or deserved punishment, or the content is a mixture of mood-incongruent and mood-congruent themes.

With catatonia: The catatonia specifier can apply to an episode of depression if catatonic features are present during most of the episode. See criteria for catatonia associated with a mental disorder (for a description of catatonia, see the chapter "Schizophrenia Spectrum and Other Psychotic Disorders" [in DSM-5]).

With peripartum onset: This specifier can be applied to the current or, if full criteria are not currently met for a major depressive episode, most recent episode of major depression if onset of mood symptoms occurs during pregnancy or in the 4 weeks following delivery.

> **Note:** Mood episodes can have their onset either during pregnancy or postpartum. Although the estimates differ according to the period of follow-up after delivery, between 3% and 6% of women will experience the onset of a major depressive episode during pregnancy or in the weeks or months following delivery. Fifty percent of "postpartum" major depressive episodes actually begin prior to delivery. Thus, these episodes are referred to collectively as *peripartum* episodes. Women with peripartum major depressive episodes often have severe anxiety and even panic attacks. Prospective studies have demonstrated that mood and anxiety symptoms during pregnancy, as well as the "baby blues," increase the risk for a postpartum major depressive episode.

> Peripartum-onset mood episodes can present either with or without psychotic features. Infanticide is most often associated with postpartum psychotic episodes that are characterized by command hallucinations to kill the infant or delusions that the infant is possessed, but psychotic symptoms can also occur in severe postpartum mood episodes without such specific delusions or hallucinations.

Postpartum mood (major depressive or manic) episodes with psychotic features appear to occur in from 1 in 500 to 1 in 1,000 deliveries and may be more common in primiparous women. The risk of postpartum episodes with psychotic features is particularly increased for women with prior postpartum mood episodes but is also elevated for those with a prior history of a depressive or bipolar disorder (especially bipolar I disorder) and those with a family history of bipolar disorders.

Once a woman has had a postpartum episode with psychotic features, the risk of recurrence with each subsequent delivery is between 30% and 50%. Postpartum episodes must be differentiated from delirium occurring in the postpartum period, which is distinguished by a fluctuating level of awareness or attention. The postpartum period is unique with respect to the degree of neuroendocrine alterations and psychosocial adjustments, the potential impact of breast-feeding on treatment planning, and the long-term implications of a history of postpartum mood disorder on subsequent family planning.

With seasonal pattern: This specifier applies to recurrent major depressive disorder.

A. There has been a regular temporal relationship between the onset of major depressive episodes in major depressive disorder and a particular time of the year (e.g., in the fall or winter).

Note: Do not include cases in which there is an obvious effect of seasonally related psychosocial stressors (e.g., regularly being unemployed every winter).

B. Full remissions (or a change from major depression to mania or hypomania) also occur at a characteristic time of the year (e.g., depression disappears in the spring).

C. In the last 2 years, two major depressive episodes have occurred that demonstrate the temporal seasonal relationships defined above and no nonseasonal major depressive episodes have occurred during that same period.

D. Seasonal major depressive episodes (as described above) substantially outnumber the nonseasonal major depressive episodes that may have occurred over the individual's lifetime.

Note: The specifier "with seasonal pattern" can be applied to the pattern of major depressive episodes in major depressive disorder, recurrent. The essential feature is the onset and remission of major depressive episodes at characteristic times of the year. In most cases, the episodes begin in fall or winter and remit in spring. Less commonly, there may be recurrent summer depressive episodes. This pattern of onset and remission of episodes must have occurred during at least a 2-year period, without any nonseasonal episodes occurring during this period. In addition, the seasonal depressive episodes must substantially outnumber any nonseasonal depressive episodes over the individual's lifetime.

This specifier does not apply to those situations in which the pattern is better explained by seasonally linked psychosocial stressors (e.g., seasonal unemployment or school schedule). Major depressive episodes that occur in a seasonal pattern are often characterized by loss of energy, hypersomnia, overeating, weight gain, and a craving for carbohydrates. It is unclear whether a seasonal pattern is more likely in recurrent major depressive disorder or in bipolar disorders. However, within the bipolar disorders group, a seasonal pattern appears to be more likely in bipolar II disorder than in bipolar I disorder. In some individuals, the onset of manic or hypo-manic episodes may also be linked to a particular season.

The prevalence of winter-type seasonal pattern appears to vary with latitude, age, and sex. Prevalence increases with higher latitudes. Age is also a strong predictor of seasonality, with younger persons at higher risk for winter depressive episodes.

Specify if:

In partial remission: Symptoms of the immediately previous major depressive epi-sode are present, but full criteria are not met, or there is a period lasting less than 2 months without any significant symptoms of a major depressive episode follow-ing the end of such an episode.

In full remission: During the past 2 months, no significant signs or symptoms of the disturbance were present.

Specify current severity:

Severity is based on the number of criterion symptoms, the severity of those symp-toms, and the degree of functional disability.

Mild: Few, if any, symptoms in excess of those required to make the diagnosis are present, the intensity of the symptoms is distressing but manageable, and the symptoms result in minor impairment in social or occupational functioning.

Moderate: The number of symptoms, intensity of symptoms, and/or functional im-pairment are between those specified for "mild" and "severe."

Severe: The number of symptoms is substantially in excess of that required to make the diagnosis, the intensity of the symptoms is seriously distressing and un-manageable, and the symptoms markedly interfere with social and occupational functioning.

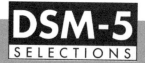

Depressive Disorders

DSM-5® Guidebook

Depressive Disorders

296.99 (F34.8)	Disruptive Mood Dysregulation Disorder
	Major Depressive Disorder, Single Episode
	Major Depressive Disorder, Recurrent Episode
300.4 (F34.1)	Persistent Depressive Disorder (Dysthymia)
625.4 (N94.3)	Premenstrual Dysphoric Disorder
	Substance/Medication-Induced Depressive Disorder
293.83 (F06.3_)	Depressive Disorder Due to Another Medical Condition
311 (F32.8)	Other Specified Depressive Disorder
311 (F32.9)	Unspecified Depressive Disorder

The major change in DSM-5 regarding mood disorders is that the DSM-IV chapter of that name has been divided into two separate chapters: one for bipolar and related disorders and the other for depressive disorders. Both diagnostic classes are reviewed in this chapter.

Mood disorders are highly prevalent, have high morbidity, and are associated with early mortality and suicide. They are among the world's most disabling illnesses, as documented in *The Global Burden of Disease* (Murray and Lopez 1996). Characterized by prominent and prolonged disturbances of mood generally inappropriate to the individual's life situation, depression and mania are considered the primary syndromes. Many symptoms occur in individuals with mood disorder, including insomnia, suicidal thoughts, anorexia, and feelings of being a burden to others in individuals with depression, and euphoria, irritability, decreased need for sleep, and hyperactivity in individuals with mania. In DSM-III, these conditions were collectively referred to as *affective disorders,* but they were renamed mood disorders for DSM-III-R. The term *mood disorder* is more appropriate because *affect* refers to fluctuating mood changes in emotional expression, whereas *mood* refers to more sustained and pervasive feeling states.

The mood disorders have been divided in many different ways over the years in attempts to identify the best classification scheme. Although that goal has been elusive, research and clinical experience both show that the fundamental symptoms of mood disorders are depressed mood, elevated mood, or an admixture of the two.

Despite having a limited number of disorders, the two DSM-5 mood disorder chapters are lengthy because of all the specifiers that can be used to provide greater detail about an individual's illness. These allow the clinician to record whether the current or most recent episode is manic, hypomanic, or depressed; whether the mood disorder is accompanied by anxious distress; whether there are mixed features, melancholic features, atypical features, psychotic features, or catatonia; whether there is rapid cycling; whether there is a peripartum onset; or whether there is a seasonal pattern.

Because mood symptoms are not specific to these diagnostic classes and are found in many other psychiatric disorders, differential diagnosis is complicated. For example, manic/hypomanic symptoms commonly occur in individuals with neurocognitive disorders or in those with schizophrenia spectrum and other psychotic disorders, whereas depression is found to some extent in individuals with disorders as wide ranging as adjustment disorders, anxiety disorders, and personality disorders. Mood symptoms are sometimes masked as complaints about insomnia, fatigue, or unexplained pain, which can further complicate the differential diagnosis.

Historically, mood disorders are among the oldest recognized psychiatric syndromes, and have been included in nearly all diagnostic classification systems through the centuries. Both depressive and bipolar conditions were included within the same category in DSM-I ("manic depressive reaction") and DSM-II ("manic-depressive illness"). All were classified as psychoses except one: mood syndromes precipitated by stressful life experience. Later, unipolar and bipolar disorders were separated in response to research showing that individuals with manic episodes have a fundamentally different course and outcome than those who experience only depression. These new concepts were reflected in the Feighner criteria (Feighner et al. 1972), the Research Diagnostic Criteria (Spitzer et al. 1975), and DSM-III. This fundamental distinction has been fully accepted by psychiatric clinicians and researchers.

The DSM-5 depressive disorders are listed in Table 1. There are two new diagnoses: disruptive mood dysregulation disorder and premenstrual dysphoric disorder. A new specifier to indicate the presence of mixed symptoms has been added across the depressive disorders. The core criterion items applied to the diagnosis major depressive disorder, as well as its 2-week duration, are unchanged from DSM-IV, although minor editing changes have been made. The Mood Disorders Work Group concluded that the major depressive disorder criteria, which were introduced in DSM-III and which had accumulated considerable research support, have held up well over the past 30 years.

One important change is the omission of the so-called bereavement exclusion. This change led to unwanted controversy whereby critics claimed it would medicalize the normal process of bereavement. In DSM-IV, major depressive episode Criterion E required that the symptoms be "not better accounted for by Bereavement." This exclusion applied to symptoms lasting less than 2 months following the death of a loved one. The change for DSM-5 was made because evidence does not support the separation of loss of a loved one from other stressors in terms of its likelihood of precipitating a major depressive episode or in terms of the relative likelihood that the symptoms will remit spontaneously. Bereavement is a severe psychosocial stressor known to precipitate major depressive episodes in vulnerable persons. Typically, when that happens, the depression begins soon after the loss. Although bereavement may be painful, most persons do not develop a major depressive episode. Those who do, however,

TABLE 1.	DSM-5 depressive disorders

Disruptive mood dysregulation disorder

Major depressive disorder, single episode

Major depressive disorder, recurrent episode

Persistent depressive disorder (dysthymia)

Premenstrual dysphoric disorder

Substance/medication-induced depressive disorder

Depressive disorder due to another medical condition

Other specified depressive disorder

Unspecified depressive disorder

typically experience more suffering, feel worthless, and may have suicidal ideation. General medical health can suffer, as can interpersonal and work function. These individuals can be at risk for "complicated grief," characterized by ruminating about the deceased person, seeking proximity to the deceased person, and striving to avoid experiences that trigger reminders of loss. Furthermore, bereavement-related depression has most of the characteristics of a major depressive episode; that is, it is most likely to occur in individuals with past personal and family history of a major depressive episode, is genetically influenced, and is associated with similar personality characteristics, patterns of comorbidity, and outcome. Finally, the symptoms associated with a bereavement-related major depressive disorder respond to antidepressant medication. Depending on the particular circumstances, the clinician observing a full depressive syndrome in an individual within the first 2 months following the death of a loved one can elect to observe rather than initiate treatment.

The coexistence within a major depressive episode of at least three manic/hypomanic symptoms insufficient to satisfy criteria for a manic/hypomanic episode is now acknowledged with the specifier "with mixed features." This change recognizes findings from family and follow-up studies that show that the presence of mixed features in an episode of major depressive disorder increases the likelihood that the illness falls within the bipolar spectrum. The presence of a full manic syndrome within a depressive episode will continue to be an exclusion criterion for a depressive disorder diagnosis, and individuals with this pattern will be considered to have a bipolar disorder.

The addition of *disruptive mood dysregulation disorder* and *premenstrual dysphoric disorder* has generated controversy, although of a different order of magnitude than that pertaining to the bereavement exclusion. Disruptive mood dysregulation disorder was created in part to address concerns about the possible overdiagnosis of bipolar disorder in children younger than 12 years who display persistent irritability and frequent episodes of extreme behavioral dyscontrol (Axelson et al. 2006). On the other hand, premenstrual dysphoric disorder was moved from Appendix B of DSM-IV ("Criteria Sets and Axes Provided for Further Study") to become a stand-alone diagnosis following a careful literature review.

There has been some controversy about the premenstrual dysphoric disorder diagnosis through the years. Some groups have felt that a disorder that focuses on the menstrual cycle may "pathologize" normal reproductive functioning. Others have believed that the disorder serves to stigmatize women's health, and perhaps implies that women would not be able to perform needed activities during the premenstrual phase of the cycle. Because the disorder is common and problematic, work group members concluded that it would be inappropriate *not* to acknowledge the condition or encourage clinicians to recognize the disorder and offer appropriate treatment.

Persistent depressive disorder (dysthymia) is new to DSM-5 and merges DSM-IV-defined chronic major depressive disorder and dysthymic disorder. Major depressive disorder may precede persistent depressive disorder, and major depressive episodes may occur during persistent depressive disorder. There is no longer a requirement that the disturbance not occur exclusively during the course of a chronic psychotic disorder, such as schizophrenia or delusional disorder (DSM-IV Criterion F). This change allows clinicians to diagnose persistent depressive disorder in persons with one of these psychotic conditions.

In summary, the depressive disorders chapter reflects refinements aimed at improving the recognition and treatment of these conditions by encouraging the clinician to record and consider specifiers that allow coverage of important information not conveyed by the categorical diagnoses themselves. New diagnoses have been added that address problems that are common and have been inadequately covered in DSM, yet are associated with significant distress and impairment, and merit recognition and special clinical management.

Disruptive Mood Dysregulation Disorder

The diagnosis of disruptive mood dysregulation disorder will help fill an important gap for children with mood dysregulation characterized by chronic, severe persistent irritability. In the past 20 years, there has been a 40-fold increase in the number of youth diagnosed with bipolar disorder. Research, however, shows that children with disruptive mood dysregulation disorder have a different outcome, gender ratio, and family history than those with bipolar disorder. Furthermore, they do not go on to develop manic or hypomanic episodes. While impaired, these children often have symptoms that meet criteria for other disruptive behavior disorders, anxiety disorders, and attention-deficit/hyperactivity disorder. The Childhood and Adolescent Disorders Work Group concluded that the best fit was with the depressive disorders.

Initially, the work group considered naming the disorder "temper dysregulation disorder" but in response to feedback chose to name it "disruptive mood dysregulation disorder." Because most of the children who meet criteria for this new disorder will also meet criteria for oppositional defiant disorder (due to overlapping symptoms), the work group decided that youth who meet criteria for both disorders should be assigned only the diagnosis of disruptive mood dysregulation disorder. This avoids the problem of having artificial comorbidity due to overlapping criteria.

Diagnostic Criteria for Disruptive Mood Dysregulation Disorder
296.99 (F34.8)

A. Severe recurrent temper outbursts manifested verbally (e.g., verbal rages) and/or behaviorally (e.g., physical aggression toward people or property) that are grossly out of proportion in intensity or duration to the situation or provocation.

B. The temper outbursts are inconsistent with developmental level.

C. The temper outbursts occur, on average, three or more times per week.

D. The mood between temper outbursts is persistently irritable or angry most of the day, nearly every day, and is observable by others (e.g., parents, teachers, peers).

E. Criteria A–D have been present for 12 or more months. Throughout that time, the individual has not had a period lasting 3 or more consecutive months without all of the symptoms in Criteria A–D.

F. Criteria A and D are present in at least two of three settings (i.e., at home, at school, with peers) and are severe in at least one of these.

G. The diagnosis should not be made for the first time before age 6 years or after age 18 years.

H. By history or observation, the age at onset of Criteria A–E is before 10 years.

I. There has never been a distinct period lasting more than 1 day during which the full symptom criteria, except duration, for a manic or hypomanic episode have been met.
Note: Developmentally appropriate mood elevation, such as occurs in the context of a highly positive event or its anticipation, should not be considered as a symptom of mania or hypomania.

J. The behaviors do not occur exclusively during an episode of major depressive disorder and are not better explained by another mental disorder (e.g., autism spectrum disorder, posttraumatic stress disorder, separation anxiety disorder, persistent depressive disorder [dysthymia]).
Note: This diagnosis cannot coexist with oppositional defiant disorder, intermittent explosive disorder, or bipolar disorder, though it can coexist with others, including major depressive disorder, attention-deficit/hyperactivity disorder, conduct disorder, and substance use disorders. Individuals whose symptoms meet criteria for both disruptive mood dysregulation disorder and oppositional defiant disorder should only be given the diagnosis of disruptive mood dysregulation disorder. If an individual has ever experienced a manic or hypomanic episode, the diagnosis of disruptive mood dysregulation disorder should not be assigned.

K. The symptoms are not attributable to the physiological effects of a substance or to another medical or neurological condition.

Criteria A and B

This item notes that the child has "severe recurrent *temper outbursts...*that are grossly out of proportion in intensity or duration to the situation or provocation" (emphasis added). Because nearly all children have temper tantrums, this criterion is needed to help distinguish ordinary tantrums from outbursts that stand apart due to their severity and regularity. Furthermore, the outbursts are inconsistent with the situation, and most parents would see these as indicating the child is out of control. Also, the outbursts are manifested verbally and/or behaviorally, such as in a tantrum, and are not consistent with the child's developmental level (i.e., the child is outside the range of the "terrible twos").

Criteria C, D, and E

The requirement that temper outbursts occur three or more times per week is somewhat arbitrary, but the point is that the outbursts occur regularly and with some frequency. Between outbursts the child's mood is persistently irritable or angry "most of the day, nearly every day." In other words, the symptoms are not just a passing phase.

These symptoms have been present for 12 or more months, during which time the child has not had at least 3 consecutive months without all of the symptoms in Criteria A–D. This item also indicates that the symptoms do not represent a temporary phase, but are pervasive and lasting.

Criterion F

The symptoms occur in at least two settings, such as at home and school. Some children seem to turn symptoms on and off at will, and this criterion separates those children in whom the symptoms seem voluntary from those who seem less likely to be able to control themselves.

Criteria G and H

This diagnosis is not made before the child is age 6 years nor after the youth turns age 18 years (Criterion G). This criterion helps to establish that the temper outbursts are not attributable to a neurodevelopmental syndrome, in which the symptoms would likely have an earlier onset, and are not attributable to adult misbehavior from an antisocial personality disorder, which is not diagnosed in persons under age 18 years.

Onset is before age 10 years (Criterion H). Again, this criterion helps guard against using the diagnosis to justify a bipolar diagnosis, which generally has an onset during adolescence or beyond.

Criteria I, J, and K

Criterion I helps separate disruptive mood dysregulation disorder from bipolar disorder by excluding individuals with symptoms that meet the full criteria for a manic or hypomanic episode for more than 1 day. Also, the item recognizes, in a note, that some "developmentally appropriate" episodes of mood elevation can occur in the context of a highly positive event or its anticipation (e.g., a birthday party, a visit to an amusement park) and should not be confused with bipolar disorder.

Criteria J and K ensure that the temper outbursts do not occur exclusively during a major depressive episode and are not better explained by another mental disorder (e.g., autism spectrum disorder), and that the symptoms are not attributable to the physiological effects of a substance or to another medical or neurological condition. It is further noted that disruptive mood dysregulation disorder cannot coexist with oppositional defiant disorder, intermittent explosive disorder, or bipolar disorder. On the other hand, it may coexist with some other mental disorders, such as major depressive disorder, attention-deficit/hyperactivity disorder, conduct disorder, and substance use disorders.

If the child's symptoms meet criteria for both disruptive mood dysregulation disorder and oppositional defiant disorder, the former diagnosis trumps the latter. Research shows that most children with disruptive mood dysregulation disorder will also have a presentation that meets criteria for oppositional defiant disorder, but the reverse is not true. Only about 15% of children with oppositional defiant disorder will have symptoms that also meet criteria for disruptive mood dysregulation disorder.

Major Depressive Episode

The syndrome major depressive episode described in DSM-III continues in DSM-5 nearly unchanged apart from editing changes, except for the bereavement exclusion and several new specifiers to help clinicians better describe an individual's episode (see "Depressive Disorders" introduction above). Major depressive disorder is the codable disorder for people with one or more major depressive episodes. Major depressive disorders are coded based on whether only a single major depressive episode has occurred or the episodes are recurrent.

Diagnostic Criteria for Major Depressive Episode

A. Five (or more) of the following symptoms have been present during the same 2-week period and represent a change from previous functioning; at least one of the symptoms is either (1) depressed mood or (2) loss of interest or pleasure.
   Note: Do not include symptoms that are clearly attributable to another medical condition.

   1. Depressed mood most of the day, nearly every day, as indicated by either subjective report (e.g., feels sad, empty, hopeless) or observation made by others (e.g., appears tearful). (**Note:** In children and adolescents, can be irritable mood.)
   2. Markedly diminished interest or pleasure in all, or almost all, activities most of the day, nearly every day (as indicated by either subjective account or observation).
   3. Significant weight loss when not dieting or weight gain (e.g., a change of more than 5% of body weight in a month), or decrease or increase in appetite nearly every day. (**Note:** In children, consider failure to make expected weight gain.)
   4. Insomnia or hypersomnia nearly every day.
   5. Psychomotor agitation or retardation nearly every day (observable by others, not merely subjective feelings of restlessness or being slowed down).
   6. Fatigue or loss of energy nearly every day.
   7. Feelings of worthlessness or excessive or inappropriate guilt (which may be delusional) nearly every day (not merely self-reproach or guilt about being sick).

    8. Diminished ability to think or concentrate, or indecisiveness, nearly every day (either by subjective account or as observed by others).

    9. Recurrent thoughts of death (not just fear of dying), recurrent suicidal ideation without a specific plan, or a suicide attempt or a specific plan for committing suicide.

B. The symptoms cause clinically significant distress or impairment in social, occupational, or other important areas of functioning.

C. The episode is not attributable to the physiological effects of a substance or to another medical condition.

Note: Criteria A–C represent a major depressive episode.

Note: Responses to a significant loss (e.g., bereavement, financial ruin, losses from a natural disaster, a serious medical illness or disability) may include the feelings of intense sadness, rumination about the loss, insomnia, poor appetite, and weight loss noted in Criterion A, which may resemble a depressive episode. Although such symptoms may be understandable or considered appropriate to the loss, the presence of a major depressive episode in addition to the normal response to a significant loss should also be carefully considered. This decision inevitably requires the exercise of clinical judgment based on the individual's history and the cultural norms for the expression of distress in the context of loss.[1]

D. The occurrence of the major depressive episode is not better explained by schizoaffective disorder, schizophrenia, schizophreniform disorder, delusional disorder, or other specified and unspecified schizophrenia spectrum and other psychotic disorders.

E. There has never been a manic episode or a hypomanic episode.

    Note: This exclusion does not apply if all of the manic-like or hypomanic-like episodes are substance-induced or are attributable to the physiological effects of another medical condition.

Coding and Recording Procedures

The diagnostic code for major depressive disorder is based on whether this is a single or recurrent episode, current severity, presence of psychotic features, and remission

---

[1] In distinguishing grief from a major depressive episode (MDE), it is useful to consider that in grief the predominant affect is feelings of emptiness and loss, while in MDE it is persistent depressed mood and the inability to anticipate happiness or pleasure. The dysphoria in grief is likely to decrease in intensity over days to weeks and occurs in waves, the so-called pangs of grief. These waves tend to be associated with thoughts or reminders of the deceased. The depressed mood of MDE is more persistent and not tied to specific thoughts or preoccupations. The pain of grief may be accompanied by positive emotions and humor that are uncharacteristic of the pervasive unhappiness and misery characteristic of MDE. The thought content associated with grief generally features a preoccupation with thoughts and memories of the deceased, rather than the self-critical or pessimistic ruminations seen in MDE. In grief, self-esteem is generally preserved, whereas in MDE feelings of worthlessness and self-loathing are common. If self-derogatory ideation is present in grief, it typically involves perceived failings vis-à-vis the deceased (e.g., not visiting frequently enough, not telling the deceased how much he or she was loved). If a bereaved individual thinks about death and dying, such thoughts are generally focused on the deceased and possibly about "joining" the deceased, whereas in MDE such thoughts are focused on ending one's own life because of feeling worthless, undeserving of life, or unable to cope with the pain of depression.

status. Current severity and psychotic features are only indicated if full criteria are currently met for a major depressive episode. Remission specifiers are only indicated if the full criteria are not currently met for a major depressive episode. Codes are as follows:

Severity/course specifier	Single episode	Recurrent episode*
Mild ([DSM-5] p. 188)	296.21 (F32.0)	296.31 (F33.0)
Moderate ([DSM-5] p. 188)	296.22 (F32.1)	296.32 (F33.1)
Severe ([DSM-5] p. 188)	296.23 (F32.2)	296.33 (F33.2)
With psychotic features** ([DSM-5] p. 186)	296.24 (F32.3)	296.34 (F33.3)
In partial remission ([DSM-5] p. 188)	296.25 (F32.4)	296.35 (F33.41)
In full remission ([DSM-5] p. 188)	296.26 (F32.5)	296.36 (F33.42)
Unspecified	296.20 (F32.9)	296.30 (F33.9)

*For an episode to be considered recurrent, there must be an interval of at least 2 consecutive months between separate episodes in which criteria are not met for a major depressive episode. The definitions of specifiers are found on the indicated pages.

**If psychotic features are present, code the "with psychotic features" specifier irrespective of episode severity.

In recording the name of a diagnosis, terms should be listed in the following order: major depressive disorder, single or recurrent episode, severity/psychotic/remission specifiers, followed by as many of the following specifiers without codes that apply to the current episode.

Specify:
With anxious distress ([DSM-5] p. 184)
With mixed features ([DSM-5] pp. 184–185)
With melancholic features ([DSM-5] p. 185)
With atypical features ([DSM-5] pp. 185–186)
With mood-congruent psychotic features ([DSM-5] p. 186)
With mood-incongruent psychotic features ([DSM-5] p. 186)
With catatonia ([DSM-5] p. 186). **Coding note:** Use additional code 293.89 (F06.1).
With peripartum onset ([DSM-5] pp. 186–187)
With seasonal pattern (recurrent episode only) ([DSM-5] pp. 187–188)

Criterion A

This item specifies that five or more of nine depressive symptoms must be present for a diagnosis of major depressive episode to be given, and at least one must be criterion A1 (depressed mood) or A2 (loss of interest or pleasure). This list has remained unchanged since DSM-III-R and contains the classic depressive symptoms recognized for centuries. Although individual symptoms are common in the general population, the fact that they cluster together over a minimum of 2 weeks to form the syndrome sets the diagnosis apart. It is important for clinicians to note that each item must be present during the 2-week period before it is counted as "present." Some symptoms that may have been present before the onset of the episode count only if they become appreciably worse during the episode. For example, some individuals have chronic insomnia that would otherwise not count unless it worsens as part of the depressive illness.

The most important symptoms are depressed mood (Criterion A1) and loss of interest or pleasure (criterion A2), and one of the two is required. Some depressed individuals will have lost the ability to describe their emotions (alexithymia) or to feel that they are depressed; others have trouble acknowledging depressed mood for cultural or other reasons. In almost all cases, the person will be able to admit to loss of interest or pleasure. Criterion A8 can be vexing because many disorders can cause poor concentration. Many individuals with mild or early forms of dementia will report memory impairment and difficulty concentrating. That said, the most important cause of these symptoms is depression and not dementia.

Suicidal thoughts or behaviors (criterion A9) are the most worrisome of the depressive symptoms, and once these are ascertained, the clinician will need to explore this symptom at greater length to determine the individual's degree of suicidality and the urgency of medical intervention.

Clinicians should note that there must be an interval of at least 2 months in which criteria are *not* met for two major depressive episodes to be considered separate and independent episodes.

Criterion B

Originally Criterion C in DSM-IV, this criterion states that depressive symptoms must cause "clinically significant distress or impairment in social, occupational, or other important areas of functioning." This criterion, added to the diagnosis in DSM-IV, is supplemented by the specifiers of mild, moderate, and severe. Although depression is perceived by most as distressing, the social and occupational impairment may manifest in a variety of ways. The individual may have poor job performance due to impaired concentration or being overly tired and therefore being inefficient at work. He or she may take too many sick days or not show up. In the social arena, the person may ignore friendships and become withdrawn; irritability may drive off remaining friends. Families may suffer because the person ignores household tasks due to lack of motivation. In severe cases, individuals may become preoccupied with thoughts of death or dying, or develop suicidal plans; some will attempt (or complete) suicide.

Criterion C

Alternative explanations for the syndrome must be eliminated during the process of differential diagnosis. Substances of abuse, medications, and other medical conditions need to be ruled out. Alcohol and other drugs are known to induce depression; in such cases, the appropriate diagnosis is substance/medication-induced depressive disorder. Likewise, medical conditions such as hypothyroidism are associated with depression and need to be ruled out as the cause; in these cases, the more appropriate diagnosis is depressive disorder due to another medical condition. These conditions will have important treatment implications.

Criterion D

The depression is not better explained by schizoaffective disorder and is not superimposed on schizophrenia, schizophreniform disorder, delusional disorder, or other specified or unspecified schizophrenia spectrum and other psychotic disorder. All of these disorders may be accompanied to some extent by the presence of depression.

Criterion E

The individual has never had a manic or a hypomanic episode. This criterion is important because it helps to separate major depressive disorder from bipolar disorder. This distinction is fundamental to the mood disorders and has important treatment implications. That said, for individuals with subsyndromal manic or hypomanic symptoms, the specifier "with mixed features" is available.

Major Depressive Disorder, Single Episode

Specifiers

The specifiers allow the clinician to describe the individual's illness in great detail, including recording whether the mood disorder is accompanied by anxious distress; whether there are mixed features, melancholic features, atypical features, psychotic features, or catatonia; and whether the depression had a peripartum onset or has a seasonal pattern. Clinicians can rate the major depressive episode as mild, moderate, or severe and as with or without psychotic features.

The DSM-IV specifier "with postpartum onset" has been changed to "with peripartum onset." This change acknowledges that half of major depressive episodes occur *prior* to delivery. The specifier is appropriate for when a major depressive episode develops during pregnancy or during the 4 weeks following delivery.

Major Depressive Disorder, Recurrent Episode

For a major depressive disorder to be considered recurrent, there must be an interval of at least 2 consecutive months between separate episodes in which criteria are not met for a major depressive episode.

Persistent Depressive Disorder (Dysthymia)

Persistent depressive disorder (dysthymia) is a chronic and persistent disturbance in mood present for at least 2 years (or at least 1 year for children and adolescents) and characterized by relatively typical depressive symptoms, such as anorexia, insomnia, decreased energy, low self-esteem, difficulty concentrating, and feelings of hopelessness. The diagnosis merges DSM-IV-defined chronic major depressive disorder and dysthymic disorder. Clinicians had trouble distinguishing the two disorders, and consolidating the disorders will make it easier to identify individuals with chronic and persistent depression.

Dysthymic disorder was introduced in DSM-III and was referred to parenthetically as depressive neurosis. Individuals with a persistent depressive disorder often develop relatively more severe major depressive episodes. When the major depressive episode clears, these individuals subsequently return to their chronic state of dysthymia. The coexistence of both mild and severe forms of depression is sometimes referred to as "double depression" because both disorders are coded.

The criteria for persistent depressive disorder are mostly unchanged from those for DSM-IV dysthymic disorder. The most important difference affects Criterion D. DSM-IV specified the *absence* of any major depressive episode in the first 2 years of the disturbance. The Mood Disorders Work Group was concerned that clinicians were unable to reliably distinguish dysthymic disorder from chronic major depressive disorder. Many clinicians were confused about the differences and tended to ignore one or the other diagnosis. Part of the confusion stems from the fact that patients are asked to recall information that most individuals are unable to retrieve. That is, does the patient recall having had in that 2-year period (that could have been decades in the past) any symptom-free periods longer than 2 months in duration, or having had 2 weeks or more in which he or she had symptoms that met criteria for a major depressive episode (in which case the patient would receive the diagnosis major depressive disorder)? These changes should help clinicians distinguish these disorders more reliably. Research also showed that there were few differences among individuals with dysthymic disorder and those with chronic major depressive disorder in symptoms, family history, or treatment response (Klein et al. 2004; McCullough et al. 2000).

Diagnostic Criteria for Persistent Depressive Disorder (Dysthymia)   **300.4 (F34.1)**

This disorder represents a consolidation of DSM-IV-defined chronic major depressive disorder and dysthymic disorder.

A. Depressed mood for most of the day, for more days than not, as indicated by either subjective account or observation by others, for at least 2 years.

   Note: In children and adolescents, mood can be irritable and duration must be at least 1 year.

B. Presence, while depressed, of two (or more) of the following:

   1. Poor appetite or overeating.
   2. Insomnia or hypersomnia.
   3. Low energy or fatigue.
   4. Low self-esteem.
   5. Poor concentration or difficulty making decisions.
   6. Feelings of hopelessness.

C. During the 2-year period (1 year for children or adolescents) of the disturbance, the individual has never been without the symptoms in Criteria A and B for more than 2 months at a time.

D. Criteria for a major depressive disorder may be continuously present for 2 years.

E. There has never been a manic episode or a hypomanic episode, and criteria have never been met for cyclothymic disorder.

F. The disturbance is not better explained by a persistent schizoaffective disorder, schizophrenia, delusional disorder, or other specified or unspecified schizophrenia spectrum and other psychotic disorder.

G. The symptoms are not attributable to the physiological effects of a substance (e.g., a drug of abuse, a medication) or another medical condition (e.g., hypothyroidism).

H. The symptoms cause clinically significant distress or impairment in social, occupational, or other important areas of functioning.

Note: Because the criteria for a major depressive episode include four symptoms that are absent from the symptom list for persistent depressive disorder (dysthymia), a very limited number of individuals will have depressive symptoms that have persisted longer than 2 years but will not meet criteria for persistent depressive disorder. If full criteria for a major depressive episode have been met at some point during the current episode of illness, they should be given a diagnosis of major depressive disorder. Otherwise, a diagnosis of other specified depressive disorder or unspecified depressive disorder is warranted.

Specify if:

With anxious distress ([DSM-5] p. 184)
With mixed features ([DSM-5] pp. 184–185)
With melancholic features ([DSM-5] p. 185)
With atypical features ([DSM-5] pp. 185–186)
With mood-congruent psychotic features ([DSM-5] p. 186)
With mood-incongruent psychotic features ([DSM-5] p. 186)
With peripartum onset ([DSM-5] pp. 186–187)

Specify if:

In partial remission ([DSM-5] p. 188)
In full remission ([DSM-5] p. 188)

Specify if:

Early onset: If onset is before age 21 years.
Late onset: If onset is at age 21 years or older.

Specify if (for most recent 2 years of persistent depressive disorder):

With pure dysthymic syndrome: Full criteria for a major depressive episode have not been met in at least the preceding 2 years.
With persistent major depressive episode: Full criteria for a major depressive episode have been met throughout the preceding 2-year period.
With intermittent major depressive episodes, with current episode: Full criteria for a major depressive episode are currently met, but there have been periods of at least 8 weeks in at least the preceding 2 years with symptoms below the threshold for a full major depressive episode.
With intermittent major depressive episodes, without current episode: Full criteria for a major depressive episode are not currently met, but there has been one or more major depressive episodes in at least the preceding 2 years.

Specify current severity:

Mild ([DSM-5] p. 188)
Moderate ([DSM-5] p. 188)
Severe ([DSM-5] p. 188)

Premenstrual Dysphoric Disorder

The Mood Disorders Work Group recommended that premenstrual dysphoric disorder receive full disorder status in DSM-5. In DSM-IV, it was included in Appendix B and, if present, was coded as depressive disorder not otherwise specified. Since the disorder was initially proposed in DSM-III-R as late luteal phase dysphoric disorder, research evidence has accumulated and shown the disorder to be prevalent and to cause significant distress and impairment. The work group felt that information on the diagnosis, treatment, and validators of the disorder had matured to the point that the disorder qualified for inclusion as an independent diagnosis.

Clinical research and epidemiological studies have shown that many women experience symptoms that begin during the luteal phase of the menstrual cycle and terminate around the onset of menses. Additionally, these studies identified a subset of women (about 2% in the community) who suffer intermittently from severe symptoms associated with the luteal phase of the menstrual cycle. Women with these symptoms have not been adequately covered in DSM. Including premenstrual dysphoric disorder helps ensure that clinicians will recognize the syndrome and that women with the disorder will receive appropriate treatment.

Diagnostic Criteria for Premenstrual Dysphoric Disorder   625.4 (N94.3)

A. In the majority of menstrual cycles, at least five symptoms must be present in the final week before the onset of menses, start to *improve* within a few days after the onset of menses, and become *minimal* or absent in the week postmenses.

B. One (or more) of the following symptoms must be present:

1. Marked affective lability (e.g., mood swings; feeling suddenly sad or tearful, or increased sensitivity to rejection).
2. Marked irritability or anger or increased interpersonal conflicts.
3. Marked depressed mood, feelings of hopelessness, or self-deprecating thoughts.
4. Marked anxiety, tension, and/or feelings of being keyed up or on edge.

C. One (or more) of the following symptoms must additionally be present, to reach a total of *five* symptoms when combined with symptoms from Criterion B above.

1. Decreased interest in usual activities (e.g., work, school, friends, hobbies).
2. Subjective difficulty in concentration.
3. Lethargy, easy fatigability, or marked lack of energy.
4. Marked change in appetite; overeating; or specific food cravings.
5. Hypersomnia or insomnia.
6. A sense of being overwhelmed or out of control.
7. Physical symptoms such as breast tenderness or swelling, joint or muscle pain, a sensation of "bloating," or weight gain.

Note: The symptoms in Criteria A–C must have been met for most menstrual cycles that occurred in the preceding year.

D. The symptoms are associated with clinically significant distress or interference with work, school, usual social activities, or relationships with others (e.g., avoidance of social activities; decreased productivity and efficiency at work, school, or home).

E. The disturbance is not merely an exacerbation of the symptoms of another disorder, such as major depressive disorder, panic disorder, persistent depressive disorder (dysthymia), or a personality disorder (although it may co-occur with any of these disorders).

F. Criterion A should be confirmed by prospective daily ratings during at least two symptomatic cycles. (**Note:** The diagnosis may be made provisionally prior to this confirmation.)

G. The symptoms are not attributable to the physiological effects of a substance (e.g., a drug of abuse, a medication, other treatment) or another medical condition (e.g., hyperthyroidism).

Substance/Medication-Induced Depressive Disorder

Substance/medication-induced depressive disorder is diagnosed when an individual's depressive symptoms have clearly resulted from the effect of a substance or from its withdrawal. Such disorders occur commonly and have been associated with particular substances, with alcohol being perhaps the most common incitant. The disorder is also frequently observed in hospital and clinic populations. The diagnostic criteria are mostly unchanged from those for substance-induced mood disorder in DSM-IV except that Criterion A has been edited to reflect the focus on depressive symptoms, as is appropriate for this chapter. Coding depends on the substance implicated as inducing the disorder. The name of the substance is included in the name of the disorder (e.g., alcohol-induced depressive disorder).

Diagnostic Criteria for Substance/Medication-Induced Depressive Disorder

A. A prominent and persistent disturbance in mood that predominates in the clinical picture and is characterized by depressed mood or markedly diminished interest or pleasure in all, or almost all, activities.

B. There is evidence from the history, physical examination, or laboratory findings of both (1) and (2):

1. The symptoms in Criterion A developed during or soon after substance intoxication or withdrawal or after exposure to a medication.

2. The involved substance/medication is capable of producing the symptoms in Criterion A.

C. The disturbance is not better explained by a depressive disorder that is not substance/medication-induced. Such evidence of an independent depressive disorder could include the following:

The symptoms preceded the onset of the substance/medication use; the symptoms persist for a substantial period of time (e.g., about 1 month) after the cessation of acute withdrawal or severe intoxication; or there is other evidence suggesting the existence of an independent non-substance/medication-induced depressive disorder (e.g., a history of recurrent non-substance/medication-related episodes).

D. The disturbance does not occur exclusively during the course of a delirium.

E. The disturbance causes clinically significant distress or impairment in social, occupational, or other important areas of functioning.

Note: This diagnosis should be made instead of a diagnosis of substance intoxication or substance withdrawal only when the symptoms in Criterion A predominate in the clinical picture and when they are sufficiently severe to warrant clinical attention.

Coding note: The ICD-9-CM and ICD-10-CM codes for the [specific substance/medication]-induced depressive disorders are indicated in the table below. Note that the ICD-10-CM code depends on whether or not there is a comorbid substance use disorder present for the same class of substance. If a mild substance use disorder is comorbid with the substance-induced depressive disorder, the 4th position character is "1," and the clinician should record "mild [substance] use disorder" before the substance-induced depressive disorder (e.g., "mild cocaine use disorder with cocaine-induced depressive disorder"). If a moderate or severe substance use disorder is comorbid with the substance-induced depressive disorder, the 4th position character is "2," and the clinician should record "moderate [substance] use disorder" or "severe [substance] use disorder," depending on the severity of the comorbid substance use disorder. If there is no comorbid substance use disorder (e.g., after a one-time heavy use of the substance), then the 4th position character is "9," and the clinician should record only the substance-induced depressive disorder.

| | | ICD-10-CM | | |
	ICD-9-CM	With use disorder, mild	With use disorder, moderate or severe	Without use disorder
Alcohol	291.89	F10.14	F10.24	F10.94
Phencyclidine	292.84	F16.14	F16.24	F16.94
Other hallucinogen	292.84	F16.14	F16.24	F16.94
Inhalant	292.84	F18.14	F18.24	F18.94
Opioid	292.84	F11.14	F11.24	F11.94
Sedative, hypnotic, or anxiolytic	292.84	F13.14	F13.24	F13.94
Amphetamine (or other stimulant)	292.84	F15.14	F15.24	F15.94
Cocaine	292.84	F14.14	F14.24	F14.94
Other (or unknown) substance	292.84	F19.14	F19.24	F19.94

Specify if (see Table 1 in the chapter "Substance-Related and Addictive Disorders" [in DSM-5] for diagnoses associated with substance class):

With onset during intoxication: If criteria are met for intoxication with the substance and the symptoms develop during intoxication.

With onset during withdrawal: If criteria are met for withdrawal from the substance and the symptoms develop during, or shortly after, withdrawal.

Depressive Disorder Due to Another Medical Condition

Some people develop depressive symptoms that are attributable to a known medical disorder. These disorders are common, particularly in hospitals and consultation-liaison services. Many physical disorders, such as hypothyroidism, are known to induce depressive disorders. The DSM-5 criteria alert clinicians to the possibility that a person's depression is induced and that a search for a medical cause may be appropriate. For that reason, this diagnosis has important treatment implications.

The diagnosis may be further specified as with depressive features, with major depressive–like episode, or with mixed features. In recording the diagnosis, the name of the other medical condition should be included in the name of the disorder (e.g., depressive disorder due to hypothyroidism, with mixed features).

Diagnostic Criteria for Depressive Disorder Due to Another Medical Condition

A. A prominent and persistent period of depressed mood or markedly diminished interest or pleasure in all, or almost all, activities that predominates in the clinical picture.

B. There is evidence from the history, physical examination, or laboratory findings that the disturbance is the direct pathophysiological consequence of another medical condition.

C. The disturbance is not better explained by another mental disorder (e.g., adjustment disorder, with depressed mood, in which the stressor is a serious medical condition).

D. The disturbance does not occur exclusively during the course of a delirium.

E. The disturbance causes clinically significant distress or impairment in social, occupational, or other important areas of functioning.

Coding note: The ICD-9-CM code for depressive disorder due to another medical condition is **293.83,** which is assigned regardless of the specifier. The ICD-10-CM code depends on the specifier (see below).

Specify if:

(F06.31) With depressive features: Full criteria are not met for a major depressive episode.

(F06.32) With major depressive–like episode: Full criteria are met (except Criterion C) for a major depressive episode.

(F06.34) With mixed features: Symptoms of mania or hypomania are also present but do not predominate in the clinical picture.

Coding note: Include the name of the other medical condition in the name of the mental disorder (e.g., 293.83 [F06.31] depressive disorder due to hypothyroidism, with depressive features). The other medical condition should also be coded and listed separately immediately before the depressive disorder due to the medical condition (e.g., 244.9 [E03.9] hypothyroidism; 293.83 [F06.31] depressive disorder due to hypothyroidism, with depressive features).

Other Specified Depressive Disorder and Unspecified Depressive Disorder

These categories replace DSM-IV's depressive disorder not otherwise specified. The category other specified depressive disorder is used when symptoms characteristic of a depressive disorder are present and cause distress or impairment but do not meet the full criteria for a more specific disorder in the class, and when the clinician chooses to communicate the reason that the presentation does not meet full criteria. The clinician is encouraged to record the specific reason (e.g., recurrent brief depression, short-duration depressive episode [4–13 days], depressive episode with insufficient symptoms).

The category unspecified depressive disorder is used when the the full criteria for a more specific disorder are not met but symptoms cause clinically significant distress or impairment, and the clinician chooses not to specify the reason the criteria are not met, or there is insufficient information to make a more specific diagnosis.

Other Specified Depressive Disorder   311 (F32.8)

This category applies to presentations in which symptoms characteristic of a depressive disorder that cause clinically significant distress or impairment in social, occupational, or other important areas of functioning predominate but do not meet the full criteria for any of the disorders in the depressive disorders diagnostic class. The other specified depressive disorder category is used in situations in which the clinician chooses to communicate the specific reason that the presentation does not meet the criteria for any specific depressive disorder. This is done by recording "other specified depressive disorder" followed by the specific reason (e.g., "short-duration depressive episode").

Examples of presentations that can be specified using the "other specified" designation include the following:

1. **Recurrent brief depression:** Concurrent presence of depressed mood and at least four other symptoms of depression for 2–13 days at least once per month (not associated with the menstrual cycle) for at least 12 consecutive months in an individual whose presentation has never met criteria for any other depressive or bipolar disorder and does not currently meet active or residual criteria for any psychotic disorder.

2. **Short-duration depressive episode (4–13 days):** Depressed affect and at least four of the other eight symptoms of a major depressive episode associated with clin-

ically significant distress or impairment that persists for more than 4 days, but less than 14 days, in an individual whose presentation has never met criteria for any other depressive or bipolar disorder, does not currently meet active or residual criteria for any psychotic disorder, and does not meet criteria for recurrent brief depression.

3. **Depressive episode with insufficient symptoms:** Depressed affect and at least one of the other eight symptoms of a major depressive episode associated with clinically significant distress or impairment that persist for at least 2 weeks in an individual whose presentation has never met criteria for any other depressive or bipolar disorder, does not currently meet active or residual criteria for any psychotic disorder, and does not meet criteria for mixed anxiety and depressive disorder symptoms.

Unspecified Depressive Disorder   **311** (F32.9)

This category applies to presentations in which symptoms characteristic of a depressive disorder that cause clinically significant distress or impairment in social, occupational, or other important areas of functioning predominate but do not meet the full criteria for any of the disorders in the depressive disorders diagnostic class. The unspecified depressive disorder category is used in situations in which the clinician chooses *not* to specify the reason that the criteria are not met for a specific depressive disorder, and includes presentations for which there is insufficient information to make a more specific diagnosis (e.g., in emergency room settings).

Key Points

- The mood disorders have been split into two chapters: "Bipolar and Related Disorders" and "Depressive Disorders."

- The wording "persistently increased goal-directed activity or energy" has been added to Criterion A for manic episode and hypomanic episode. This should make explicit the requirement that this hallmark symptom of bipolar I or II disorder needs to be present for the diagnosis to be made.

- The diagnosis of bipolar I disorder, most recent episode mixed, which required criteria for both mania and major depressive episode to be met simultaneously, has been deleted. Instead, a "with mixed features" specifier has been added that can be applied to a manic episode or a hypomanic episode when depressive features are present.

- With the depressive disorders, an important change is the omission of the bereavement exclusion that applied in DSM-IV to depressive symptoms lasting less than 2 months following the death of a loved one. This change was made because evidence does not support the separation of loss of a loved one from other stressors in terms of its likelihood of precipitating a major depressive episode.

- Disruptive mood dysregulation disorder is new to the depressive disorders and describes the presentation of children with persistent irritability and behavioral dyscontrol. This change should help reduce the problem of overdiagnosis of bipolar disorder in children and adolescents.

- Persistent depressive disorder (dysthymia) is new and merges DSM-IV-defined chronic major depressive disorder and dysthymic disorder. Clinicians had trouble distinguishing the two disorders.

- Premenstrual dysphoric disorder has been elevated to a stand-alone diagnosis. The diagnosis applies to the presentation of women who develop a cluster of depressive symptoms in association with their menstrual cycle.

References

Axelson D, Birmaher B, Strober M, et al: Phenomenology of children and adolescents with bipolar spectrum disorders. Arch Gen Psychiatry 63:1139–1148, 2006

Feighner JP, Robins E, Guze SB, et al: Diagnostic criteria for use in psychiatric research. Arch Gen Psychiatry 26:57–63, 1972

Klein DN, Shankman SA, Lewinsohn PM, et al: Family study of chronic depression in a community sample of young adults. Am J Psychiatry 161:646–653, 2004

McCullough JP Jr, Klein DN, Keller MB, et al: Comparison of DSM-III-R chronic major depression and major depression superimposed on dysthymia (double depression): validity of the distinction. J Abnorm Psychol 109:419–427, 2000

Murray CJL, Lopez AD: The Global Burden of Disease. Boston, MA, Harvard University Press, 1996

Spitzer RL, Endicott J, Robins E: Research diagnostic criteria (RDC). New York, Biometrics Research, New York State Psychiatric Institute, 1975

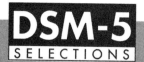

Depressive Disorders

DSM-5® Clinical Cases

Introduction

John W. Barnhill, M.D.

Depression is one of the most commonly used words in psychiatry, and it is also one of the most ambiguous. As a symptom it can mean sadness, but as a diagnosis it can be applied to people who deny feeling sad. Depressed mood is a common, normal human experience, but it can also reflect a seriously debilitating, distressing, and potentially fatal condition. Depression can present in multiple ways, with many potential comorbidities, precipitants, and reliably associated symptoms.

DSM-5 makes use of available evidence to fine-tune multiple diagnostic categories. For example, although bipolar disorder has historically been viewed as "manic depression," and therefore as a subset of depression, it has become increasingly clear that while bipolar and depressive disorders have similarities, they also have substantive differences in regard to clinical presentation, family history, longitudinal course, and treatment. For these reasons, bipolar disorder has been moved into its own chapter in DSM-5. The overlap persists, however, and the depressive and bipolar disorder chapters go into detail in an effort to distinguish the sometimes subtle differences between diagnoses.

Major depressive disorder remains the archetypal depression, and its diagnostic criteria are essentially unchanged in DSM-5. The diagnosis still hinges on the assessment of clinical presentation (five of nine symptoms), history (persistence greater than 2 weeks), and relevance (significant distress or impairment). To further subdivide this broad category, DSM-5 provides specifiers that distinguish the episode based on severity and recurrence as well as the presence of such factors as melancholia, psychotic features, and catatonia. A particularly useful change within DSM-5 is the delinkage of psychosis and severity, so the clinician can accurately describe people whose depressive symptoms are, say, moderate, but who have an associated psychosis.

The chapter on depressive disorders also includes several changes that have been the subject of significant scrutiny. The so-called bereavement exclusion has perhaps been the most discussed. It is widely understood that mourning the death of a loved one is a normal human reaction, and DSM-IV clarified that a 2-month period of bereavement was necessary before a major depression diagnosis could generally be made. Evidence indicates, however, that the vast majority of grieving people do not develop the symptoms of major depression. In other words, major depression that occurs in the context of bereavement is not a "normal" reaction. The suffering of major depression tends to include more intense feelings of guilt, worthlessness, and suicidality, for example, and the functional decline is more intense. Furthermore, individuals who develop major depressive symptoms soon after the death of a loved one have elevated rates of depression in their personal and family histories, tend to have a worse prognosis, and tend to respond to antidepressant medications. In other words, individuals who develop all the characteristics of a major depression following the death of a loved one are similar to people who develop major depression following any other serious stress and deserve the same level of clinical attention.

Just as grief is a normal reaction to loss, temper tantrums are a normal part of childhood. There are, however, children whose low frustration tolerance and behavioral dyscontrol transcend those of normal human experience; their affective dysregulation not only is distressing to their parents, teachers, and classmates, but also is upsetting to the affected children and threatens to derail their normal development. A second change in DSM-5 is that these children are categorized as having disruptive mood dysregulation disorder (DMDD). Controversies about DMDD fall into two camps. In the first, there is concern that DSM-5 might pathologize normal childhood experience. In the second, there is a view that such behavior is more accurately described within the bipolar spectrum of disorders. Evidence indicates, however, that DMDD does describe a cluster of prepubescent children who are significantly distressed and dysfunctional and who are at risk for a lifetime of difficulty. Furthermore, it appears that DMDD is not simply a childhood form of bipolar disorder. In fact, DMDD is much more likely to convert in adulthood to a depressive or anxiety disorder than to a bipolar disorder.

A third change is the shift of premenstrual dysphoric disorder (PMDD) from the appendix into the main text of DSM-5. Just as DMDD does not refer to average expectable "temper tantrums," PMDD does not describe the transient, mild symptoms that are commonly described as "premenstrual syndrome." Instead, PMDD describes a robust cluster of symptoms that cause persistent, significant debility and distress.

Concerns have been raised that these three changes can lead to the pathologizing of normal human experience and, secondarily, to the excess use of psychiatric medication. The field of psychiatry should indeed recognize both the limitations of current evidence and the external forces that might try to influence the field for their own reward. At the same time, evidence does indicate that these three diagnoses reflect three clusters of people who are suffering and significantly dysfunctional. It is also true that people meeting these criteria are already seeking psychiatric help, and that the development of rigorous diagnostic criteria allows for replicable research into effective biopsychosocial interventions.

Suggested Readings

Keller MB, Coryell WH, Endicott J, et al (eds): Clinical Guide to Depression and Bipolar Disorder: Findings From the Collaborative Depression Study. Washington, DC, American Psychiatric Publishing, 2013

Kramer P: Against Depression. New York, Penguin, 2006

Maj M: Clinical judgment and the DSM-5 diagnosis of major depression. World Psychiatry 12(2):89–91, 2013. Available at: http://www.ncbi.nlm.nih.gov/pmc/articles/PMC3683250. Accessed August 29, 2013.

Case 1: Moody and Irritable

William C. Wood, M.D.

Wyatt was a 12-year-old-boy referred by his psychiatrist to an adolescent partial hospitalization program because of repeated conflicts that have frightened both classmates and family members.

According to his parents, Wyatt was generally moody and irritable, with frequent episodes of being "a raging monster." It had become almost impossible to set limits. Most recently, Wyatt had smashed a closet door to gain access to a video game that had been withheld to encourage him to do homework. At school, Wyatt was noted to have a hair-trigger temper, and he had recently been suspended for punching another boy in the face after losing a chess match.

Wyatt had been an extremely active young boy, running "all the time." He was also a "sensitive kid" who constantly worried that things might go wrong. His tolerance for frustration had been less than that of his peers, and his parents quit taking him shopping because he would predictably become distraught whenever they did not buy him whatever toys he wanted.

Grade school reports indicated fidgetiness, wandering attention, and impulsivity. When Wyatt was 10 years old, a child psychiatrist diagnosed him as having attention-deficit/hyperactivity disorder (ADHD), combined type. Wyatt was referred to a behavioral therapist and started taking methylphenidate, with an improvement in symptoms. By fourth grade, his moodiness became more pronounced and persistent. He was generally surly, complaining that life was "unfair." Wyatt and his parents began their daily limit-setting battles at breakfast while he delayed getting ready for school, and then—by evening—continued their arguments about homework, video games, and bedtime. These arguments often included Wyatt screaming and throwing nearby objects. By the time he reached sixth grade, his parents were tired and his siblings avoided him.

According to Wyatt's parents, he had no problems with appetite, and although they fought about when he would go to bed, he did not appear to have a sleep disturbance. He appeared to find pleasure in his usual activities, maintained good energy, and had no history of elation, grandiosity, or decreased need for sleep lasting more than a day. Although they described him as "moody, isolated, and lonely," his parents did not see him as depressed. They denied any history of hallucinations, abuse, trauma, suicidality, homicidality, a wish to self-harm, or any premeditated wish to harm others. He and his parents denied he had ever used alcohol or drugs. His medical history was unremarkable. His family history was notable for anxiety and depression in the father, alcoholism in the paternal grandparents, and possible untreated ADHD in the mother.

On interview, Wyatt was mildly anxious yet easy to engage. His body twisted back and forth as he sat in the chair. In reviewing his temper outbursts and physical aggression, Wyatt said, "It's like I can't help myself. I don't mean to do these things. But when I get mad, I don't think about any of that. It's like my mind goes blank." When asked how he felt about his outbursts, Wyatt looked very sad and said earnestly, "I hate when I'm that way." If he could change three things in his life, Wyatt replied, "I would have more friends, I would do better in school, and I would stop getting mad so much."

Diagnoses

- Disruptive mood dysregulation disorder
- Attention-deficit/hyperactivity disorder, combined presentation

Discussion

Wyatt's psychiatrist has referred him to an adolescent partial hospitalization program because of persistent irritability and severe recurrent temper outbursts.

In assessing this 12-year-old boy, it would be important to attend to the quality, severity, frequency, and duration of the outbursts. Are they outside the range of "developmentally normal" children? What are the provocations? Do the outbursts occur at home, at school, with peers, or in more than one setting? How are they affecting his life? What is this boy's general mood between the outbursts? Do the outbursts reflect a lack of control over his emotional reactions, or are they a behavior calculated to achieve an intended outcome? At what age did these emotional and/or behavioral outbursts begin? Are there corresponding neurovegetative depressive symptoms? Has he ever exhibited manic-like symptoms such as grandiosity, decreased need for sleep, pressured speech, or racing thoughts? If so, have these symptoms persisted long enough to meet criteria for a manic episode? Does he abuse substances? Has he ever experienced psychotic symptoms such as paranoia, delusions, or hallucinations of any kind?

In Wyatt's case, his intense irritability appears to be persistent, while his outbursts tend to be extreme and incongruent with his overall developmental level. They are clearly interfering with all aspects of his life. He does not appear to be in control of his behavior, and his irritability and outbursts are not bringing him anything positive; in fact, the three things he says he would most like to change are specifically related to either the symptom ("stop getting mad so much") or the consequences of his symptoms ("have more friends" and "do better in school"). These symptoms have been worsening since grade school. He lacks prominent neurovegetative symptoms of depression, and there is no history of mania, psychosis, or substance abuse. Therefore, he meets criteria for disruptive mood dysregulation disorder (DMDD), a new diagnosis in DSM-5 that is listed among the depressive disorders.

The core feature of DMDD is chronic, severe, persistent irritability that is incongruent with a child's developmental stage and is causing significant impairment. DSM-5 defines this core feature as having two prominent clinical manifestations: frequent severe temper outbursts (verbal or behavioral) and chronic, persistently irritable or angry mood that is present between the severe temper outbursts.

Although some of the symptoms of DMDD can overlap with those of other diagnoses, DMDD does appear to represent a cluster of young people whose symptom profiles differ from those of other DSM-5 diagnoses and transcend age-congruent "temper tantrums." For example, bipolar disorder can also lead to interpersonal conflicts and irritability. However, children and adolescents with DMDD do not exhibit other core symptoms of mania, such as decreased need for sleep, pressured speech, mood cycling, and racing thoughts that persist for several days at a time. Disruptive behavior disorders such as oppositional defiant disorder, intermittent explosive disorder, and conduct disorder differ from DMDD in that they are not marked by intense irritability that persists between outbursts.

By DSM-5 definition, DMDD cannot coexist with bipolar disorder or with either oppositional defiant disorder or intermittent explosive disorder. If the patient has ever had a manic episode, a diagnosis of bipolar disorder supersedes a DMDD diagnosis. If the patient meets criteria for intermittent explosive disorder or oppositional defiant disorder but also meets criteria for DMDD, the patient should only be diagnosed with DMDD.

DMDD can be comorbid with a variety of other diagnoses. For example, Wyatt presents with long-standing problems with attention and anxiety. When in grade school, he was diagnosed with ADHD, combined type, which indicates that he met most criteria in both ADHD categories: attention and hyperactivity/impulsivity. Wyatt is also noted to be a chronic worrier. Although this was not explored at length in the history, he may well qualify for an anxiety disorder.

It will be important to follow Wyatt longitudinally. The goal, of course, is to employ the most parsimonious diagnostic assessment and treatment plan, but these can change in the context of Wyatt's overall development. As an adolescent with a diagnosis of DMDD, he will continue to be at risk for a variety of comorbid psychiatric conditions, including other mood, anxiety, and substance use disorders.

Suggested Readings

Axelson D, Findling RL, Fristad MA, et al: Examining the proposed disruptive mood dysregulation disorder diagnosis in children in the Longitudinal Assessment of Manic Symptoms study. J Clin Psychiatry 73(10):1342–1350, 2012

Copeland WE, Angold A, Costello EJ, et al: Prevalence, comorbidity, and correlates of DSM-5 proposed disruptive mood dysregulation disorder. Am J Psychiatry 170(2):173–179, 2013

Leibenluft E: Severe mood dysregulation, irritability, and the diagnostic boundaries of bipolar disorder in youths. Am J Psychiatry 168(2):129–142, 2011

Margulies DM, Weintraub S, Basile J, et al: Will disruptive mood dysregulation disorder reduce false diagnosis of bipolar disorder in children? Bipolar Disord 14(5):488–496, 2012

Mikita N, Stringaris A: Mood dysregulation. Eur Child Adolesc Psychiatry 22 (suppl 1):S11–S16, 2013

Wozniak J, Biederman J, Kiely K, et al: Mania-like symptoms suggestive of childhood-onset bipolar disorder in clinically referred children. J Am Acad Child Adolesc Psychiatry 34(7):867–876, 1995

Case 2: Postpartum Sadness

Kimberly A. Yonkers, M.D.
Heather B. Howell, M.S.W.

Yvonne Perez was a 23-year-old woman who presented for an outpatient psychiatric evaluation 2 weeks after giving birth to her second child. She was referred by her breast-feeding nurse, who was concerned about the patient's depressed mood, flat affect, and fatigue.

Ms. Perez said she had been worried and unenthusiastic since finding out she was pregnant. She and her husband had planned to wait a few years before having another child, and her husband had made it clear that he would have preferred that she terminate the pregnancy, an option she would not consider because of her religion. He had also been upset that she was "too tired" to do paid work outside of the home during her pregnancy. She had then become increasingly dysphoric, hopeless, and overwhelmed after the delivery. Breast-feeding was not going well, and she had begun to believe her baby was "rejecting me" by refusing her breast, spitting up her milk, and crying. Her baby had become very colicky, so she felt forced to hold him most of the day. She wondered whether she deserved this difficulty because she had not wanted the pregnancy.

Her husband was gone much of the time for work, and she found it very difficult to take care of the new baby and her lively and demanding 16-month-old daughter. She slept little, felt constantly tired, cried often, and worried about how she was going to get through the day. Her mother-in-law had just arrived to help her care for the children.

Ms. Perez was an English-speaking Hispanic woman who had worked in a coffee shop until midway through her first pregnancy, almost 2 years earlier. She had been raised in a supportive home by her parents and a large extended family. She had moved to a different region of the country when her husband had been transferred for work, and she had no relatives nearby. Although no one in her family had seen a psychiatrist, several family members appeared to have been depressed. She had no prior psychiatric history or treatment. She denied illicit drug or alcohol use. She had smoked for several years but stopped when she was pregnant with her first child. Ms. Perez had a history of asthma. Aside from a multivitamin with iron, she took no medications.

On mental status examination, Ms. Perez was a casually dressed, cooperative young woman. She made some eye contact, but her eyes tended to drop to the floor when she spoke. Her speech was fluent but slow, with increased latency when answering questions. The tone of her speech was flat. She endorsed low mood, and her affect was constricted. She denied thoughts of suicide and homicide. She also denied any hallucinations and delusions, although she had considered whether the current situation was punishment for not wanting the child. She was fully oriented and could register three objects but only recalled one after 5 minutes. Her intelligence was average. Her insight and judgment were fair to good.

Diagnosis

- Major depressive disorder, single episode, moderate severity, without psychotic features, with peripartum onset

Discussion

Ms. Perez presents with low mood, poor energy and sleep, psychomotor retardation, guilt, and poor concentration. The case report does not address her appetite, her ability to find pleasure, or the presence of thoughts about death, but she clearly has more than the required five of nine symptoms to meet criteria for a DSM-5 diagnosis of major depression. Contributors include the recent delivery, a family history of depression, and multiple psychosocial stressors, including a lack of support from her husband, financial troubles, a colicky baby, a rambunctious toddler, and geographic distance from her family of origin.

The case report is not clear, but it appears that Ms. Perez had significant depressive symptoms throughout the pregnancy and that she was referred to a psychiatrist at this particular time not because she was dramatically more depressed but because she was seen by a health professional, the breast-feeding nurse. If Ms. Perez became depressed only after delivery, she may not have had symptoms for the 2 weeks that are required for a major depression. In that case, adjustment disorder with depressed mood might be a more appropriate diagnosis. A postpartum onset might also increase her risk of having bipolar disorder rather than unipolar depressive disorder. Arguing against a diagnosis of bipolar disorder in this patient is the lack of any known manic or psychotic symptoms as well as the absence of a history of mood episodes or a family history of bipolar disorder. Still, the fact that she experienced precipitous worsening after delivery would increase the risk that she might develop bipolar disorder.

If Ms. Perez had low mood throughout the pregnancy and a brief worsening after delivery, then her symptoms might be viewed as a minor depressive disorder (in DSM-5, diagnosed as other specified depressive disorder) rather than major depressive disorder.

From the available history, it appears more likely that Ms. Perez had significant depressive symptoms throughout the pregnancy. She said she felt "worried and unenthusiastic" and had felt "too tired" to work. This would not be an unusual depression trajectory, because half of women who are found to be depressed after delivery were already depressed during pregnancy. DSM-5 now includes a specifier, "with peripartum onset," for women who develop a mood disorder during or soon after a pregnancy. Ms. Perez also worries that her infant is rejecting her and that her current situation is a punishment. These appear to be overvalued ideas rather than delusions, but it would be reasonable to do ongoing assessments for psychotic thinking.

It is also important to do a suicide risk assessment for everyone with symptoms of a major depression. Ms. Perez denies such symptoms, but it would be potentially useful to explore any thoughts she might have of death, of her family being better off without her, and of her children being better off dead.

The depressive subtype is important to clarify because many women with postpartum subsyndromal depressive symptoms improve spontaneously within weeks of delivery. This can occur even in the absence of formal treatment. For this reason, and because many women wish to continue breast-feeding, an initial treatment approach may be psychotherapeutic rather than pharmacological.

Suggested Readings

Munk-Olsen T, Laursen TM, Meltzer-Brody S, et al: Psychiatric disorders with postpartum onset: possible early manifestations of bipolar affective disorders. Arch Gen Psychiatry
69(4):428–434, 2012
O'Hara MW, Swain AM: Rates and risk of postpartum depression: a meta-analysis. Int Rev
Psychiatry 8:37–54, 1996
Yonkers KA, Ramin SM, Rush AJ, et al: Onset and persistence of postpartum depression in an
inner-city maternal health clinic system. Am J Psychiatry 158(11):1856–1863, 2001
Yonkers KA, Wisner KL, Stewart DE, et al: The management of depression during pregnancy:
a report from the American Psychiatric Association and the American College of Obstetri-
cians and Gynecologists. Gen Hosp Psychiatry 31(5):403–413, 2009

Case 3: Grief and Depression

Richard A. Friedman, M.D.

Andrew Quinn, a 60-year-old businessman, returned to see his longtime psychiatrist 2 weeks after the death of his 24-year-old son. The young man, who had struggled with major depression and substance abuse, had been found surrounded by several emptied pill bottles and an incoherent suicide note.

Mr. Quinn had been very close to his troubled son, and he immediately felt crushed, like his life had lost its meaning. In the ensuing 2 weeks, he had constant images of his son and was "obsessed" with how he might have prevented the substance abuse and suicide. He worried that he had been a bad father and that he had spent too much time on his own career and too little time with his son. He felt constantly sad, withdrew from his usual social life, and was unable to concentrate on his work. Although he had never previously drunk more than a few glasses of wine per week, he increased his alcohol intake to half a bottle of wine each night. At that time, his psychiatrist told him that he was struggling with grief and that such a reaction was normal. They agreed to meet for support and to assess the ongoing clinical situation.

Mr. Quinn returned to see his psychiatrist weekly. By the sixth week after the suicide, his symptoms had worsened. Instead of thinking about what he might have done differ-ently, he became preoccupied that he should have been the one to die, not his young son. He continued to have trouble falling asleep, but he also tended to awake at 4:30 A.M. and just stare at the ceiling, feeling overwhelmed with fatigue, sadness, and feelings of worthlessness. These symptoms improved during the day, but he also felt a persistent and uncharacteristic loss of self-confidence, sexual interest, and enthusiasm. He asked his psychiatrist whether he still had normal grief or had a major depression.

Mr. Quinn had a history of two prior major depressive episodes that improved with psychotherapy and antidepressant medication, but no significant depressive episodes since his 30s. He denied a history of alcohol or substance abuse. Both of his parents had been "depressive" but without treatment. No one in the family had previously committed suicide.

Diagnosis

• Major depressive disorder

Discussion

In the weeks after his son's suicide, Mr. Quinn developed sadness, insomnia, social withdrawal, diminished pleasure in activities, and poor concentration. This symptom cluster is typical of grief, recognized by both the lay public and medical professionals as a normal human reaction to the death of a loved one.

At the first meeting with the psychiatrist, Mr. Quinn demonstrated multiple symptoms that are typically found in a major depression, but his symptoms at that point appeared to be better conceptualized as normal bereavement. Such a view is supported by the fact that grief—despite causing distress and dysfunction—typically runs its course within 2–6 months without specific clinical attention.

DSM-IV acknowledged the normalcy of grief by mandating that a diagnosis of major depressive disorder (MDD) be deferred for 2 months unless the clinical presentation was characterized by unusually severe symptoms such as suicidal ideation or psychosis. Also, DSM-IV included a bereavement exclusion for a good reason: although uncomplicated grief can be painful, it is short-lived and benign, and does not severely impair function or increase the risk of suicide as does major depression.

Some people, however, do develop an autonomous mood disorder after the death of a loved one, as well as after other traumas, such as financial ruin, losses from a natural disaster, or a serious medical illness or disability. Severely distressing and causing serious impairment, such mood syndromes warrant clinical attention prior to reaching DSM-IV's 2-month cutoff, during which time most depressive symptoms are attributable to bereavement.

Because of the significant symptomatic overlap between bereavement and major depression, the difficulty in predicting which symptoms will persist or intensify and which will improve on their own, and the uncertainty over what is psychologically different between the loss of a loved one and, for example, the loss of a home due to a natural disaster, there has been significant attention paid to fine-tuning the differences between MDD and bereavement.

This redefinition of the bereavement exclusion was one of the most controversial of all the proposed changes in DSM-5. Not only does it involve a universal human experience—grief—but it raises a core concern about psychiatry, both from within and outside the field: what is normal? Various DSM-5 drafts were debated, and many people (including myself) worried that removal of the bereavement exclusion would medicalize normal grief and erroneously label healthy people with a psychiatric diagnosis.

As ultimately published, DSM-5 makes fairly modest changes, but the controversies embedded in the bereavement exclusion are relevant to this case.

In assessing depressive symptoms in the context of grief, DSM-5 suggests that Mr. Quinn's psychiatrist use her clinical judgment in differentiating between the emptiness and loss that are typical of grief and the persistently depressed mood, anhedonia, and pessimistic ruminations that are more typical of MDD. In grief, the dysphoria should gradually attenuate over weeks, though interrupted perhaps by pangs of grief that tend to focus on the deceased. The depressive symptoms of MDD are less exclusively connected to the deceased, less likely to be interrupted by positive emotions and humor, and more likely to be accompanied by self-criticism and feelings of worthlessness.

When Mr. Quinn was seen 2 weeks after the suicide, his psychiatrist rightly viewed his reaction as within the bounds of a normal grief reaction. At the same time, Mr. Quinn had risk factors for MDD that are often not present in people who are grieving. He has a personal history of two prior major depressive episodes, his family history is positive for depression in both parents, and his son may also have been depressed. All of these factors increase Mr. Quinn's likelihood of developing MDD in the context of the death of his son.

While deferring a diagnosis of MDD, the psychiatrist continued to meet weekly with Mr. Quinn. After about 6 weeks, his symptoms had worsened, both in terms of intensity and the development of cognitive and neurovegetative symptoms, making the diagnosis of major depression clear. The DSM-IV 2-month bereavement exclusion might have encouraged Mr. Quinn's psychiatrist to delay a diagnosis of MDD for another several weeks, until the 2-month mark had been reached. DSM-5, by contrast, does not specifically limit the use of an MDD diagnosis during the time frame between 2 weeks and 2 months. For Mr. Quinn, this shift likely means that he would more quickly receive a diagnosis of MDD under DSM-5.

Experts in favor of the removal of the 2-month bereavement exclusion might be reassured by Mr. Quinn's clinical assessment. With worsening symptoms and a strong personal and family history of depression, Mr. Quinn probably warrants specific clinical attention. Such concern is understandable, particularly because 10%–20% of bereaved individuals go on to experience a syndrome of complicated grief, characterized by an intense longing for and disturbing preoccupation with the deceased and a sense of anger and disbelief over the death. Furthermore, only half of individuals with major depression in the general population and 33% of depressed patients in the primary care setting receive any treatment for depression.

For most grieving people, however, their depressive symptoms do not indicate a major depression. For example, a study using data from the National Epidemiologic Survey on Alcohol and Related Conditions showed that subjects who had a bereavement-related depressive syndrome at baseline were no more likely over a 3-year follow-up period to have a major depressive episode than were those who had no lifetime history of major depression at baseline. These data confirm the widely held view that for most people, grief resolves on its own.

DSM-5 acknowledges this reality and urges clinicians to use their judgment when trying to distinguish between clinical depression and grief. It remains to be seen whether this lowering of the barrier to a major depressive diagnosis will help in identifying patients who warrant clinical attention—or encourage the medicalizing of grief. In the meantime, clinicians should continue to recognize that although grief can sometimes trigger major depression, grief itself is an entirely normal emotional response to loss that requires no treatment.

Suggested Readings

Friedman RA: Grief, depression and the DSM-5. N Engl J Med 366(20):1855–1857, 2012

Kessler RC, Berglund P, Demler O, et al: The epidemiology of major depressive disorder: results from the National Comorbidity Survey Replication (NCS-R). JAMA 289(23):3095–3105, 2003

Mojtabai R: Bereavement-related depressive episodes: characteristics, 3-year course, and implications for the DSM-5. Arch Gen Psychiatry 68(9):920–928, 2011

Shear K, Frank E, Houck PR, et al: Treatment of complicated grief: a randomized controlled trial. JAMA 293(21):2601–2608, 2005

Case 4: Lost Interest in Life

Anthony J. Rothschild, M.D.

Barbara Reiss was a 51-year-old white woman who was brought to the emergency room by her husband with the chief complaint "I feel like killing myself."

Ms. Reiss had begun to "lose interest in life" about 4 months earlier. During that time, she reported depression every day for most of the day. Symptoms had been worsening for months. She had lost 9 pounds (current weight=105 pounds) without dieting because she did not feel like eating. She had trouble falling asleep almost every night and woke at 3:00 A.M. several mornings per week (she normally woke at 6:30 A.M.). She had diminished energy, concentration, and ability to do her administrative job at a dog food processing plant. She was convinced that she had made a mistake that would lead to the deaths of thousands of dogs. She expected that she would soon be arrested, and would rather kill herself than go to prison.

Her primary care physician had recognized the patient's depressed mood 1 week earlier and had prescribed sertraline and referred her for a psychiatric evaluation.

Ms. Reiss denied previous psychiatric history. One sister suffered from depression. Ms. Reiss denied any history of hypomania or mania. She typically drank a glass of wine with dinner and had started drinking a second glass before bed in hopes of getting a night's sleep. She had been married to her husband for 20 years, and they had three school-age children. She had been employed with her current company for 13 years. She denied illicit drug use.

The physical examination performed by the primary care physician 1 week earlier was noncontributory. All laboratory testing was normal, including complete blood count, electrolytes, blood urea nitrogen, creatinine, calcium, glucose, thyroid function tests, folate, and vitamin B_{12}.

On mental status examination, Ms. Reiss was cooperative and exhibited psychomotor agitation. She answered most questions with short answers, often simply saying "yes" or "no." Speech was of a normal rate and tone, without tangentiality or circumstantiality. She denied having hallucinations or unusual thoughts. She described the mistakes she believed she had made at work and insisted that she would soon be arrested for the deaths of dogs, but she insisted this was all true and not "a delusion." Recent and remote memory were grossly intact.

Diagnosis

• Major depressive disorder, single episode, moderate, with psychotic features

Discussion

The core criteria for the diagnosis of an episode of major depressive disorder (MDD) and the requisite duration of at least 2 weeks have not changed from DSM-IV to DSM-5. Ms. Reiss has exhibited all nine of the symptomatic criteria for major depression: depressed mood, loss of interest or pleasure, weight loss, insomnia, psychomotor agitation, loss of energy, excessive guilt, trouble concentrating, and thoughts of death. Only five are necessary for a major depression diagnosis.

Before a depression diagnosis is made, a medical cause should be ruled out. A recent medical examination was noncontributory, and there is no indication that Ms. Reiss even has a medical comorbidity, much less one that could cause a depression. It is also important to explore the possibility of bipolar disorder. The case report makes no mention of such symptoms as pressured speech or risk taking, but manic symptoms can sometimes be missed, and a bipolar disorder diagnosis would significantly affect treatment. The patient reports two nightly glasses of wine, which is unlikely to be contributory. If she is significantly underestimating her alcohol intake, however, she would be at risk for alcohol-induced depressive disorder. Multiple medications and substances of abuse can also cause serious depression and psychosis. Collateral history might be helpful, as would a toxicology screen.

Ms. Reiss also exhibits psychotic symptoms (delusions) in the context of MDD. New to DSM-5 is the separation of psychotic features from the major depression severity rating. In other words, MDD with psychotic features is not inevitably considered "severe." Ms. Reiss's psychotic symptoms would be classified as mood congruent because the content of her delusions is consistent with the typical depressive themes of inadequacy, guilt, disease, death, nihilism, and/or deserved punishment. Notably, in DSM-5, a hierarchy giving precedence to mood-incongruent features is being introduced to allow classification of cases in which mood-congruent and mood-incongruent psychoses coexist.

Psychotic features can often be missed in major depression. Although Ms. Reiss's delusions about killing dogs appear to have been spontaneously reported and are unlikely to be true, many patients are more guarded and do not easily give up such information. Furthermore, fixed, false beliefs that are not bizarre can sound reasonable to the clinician. One way to approach this issue with patients is to avoid use of words such as *psychosis* or *delusional* and instead ask about "irrational worries."

Suggested Readings

Maj M, Pirozzi R, Magliano L, et al: Phenomenology and prognostic significance of delusions in major depressive disorder: a 10-year prospective follow-up study. J Clin Psychiatry 68(9):1411–1417, 2007

Rothschild AJ (ed): Clinical Manual for the Diagnosis and Treatment of Psychotic Depression. Washington, DC, American Psychiatric Publishing, 2009

Rothschild AJ, Winer J, Flint AJ, et al: Missed diagnosis of psychotic depression at 4 academic medical centers. J Clin Psychiatry 69(8):1293–1296, 2008

Case 5: Despair

Cheryl Munday, Ph.D.
Jamie Miller Abelson, M.S.W.
James Jackson, Ph.D.

Crystal Smith, a 33-year-old African American homemaker, came to an outpatient clinic seeking "someone to talk to" about feelings of despair that had intensified over the previous 8–10 months. She was particularly upset about marital conflict and an uncharacteristic mistrust of her in-laws.

Ms. Smith said she had begun to wake before dawn, feeling down and tearful. She had difficulty getting out of bed and completing her usual household activities. At times, she felt guilty for not being her "usual self." At other times, she became easily irritated with her husband and her in-laws for minor transgressions. She had previously relied on her mother-in-law to assist with the children, but she no longer entirely trusted her with that responsibility. That worry, in combination with her insomnia and fatigue, made it very difficult for Ms. Smith to get her children to school on time. In the past few months, she had lost 13 pounds without dieting. She denied current suicidal ideation, saying she "would never do something like that," but acknowledged having thought that she "should just give up" and that she "would be better off dead."

Two months previously, Ms. Smith had seen a psychiatrist for several weeks and received fluoxetine. She reluctantly gave it a try, discontinuing it quickly because it made her feel tired. She had also dropped out of therapy, indicating that the psychiatrist did not seem to understand her.

Ms. Smith lived with her husband of 13 years and two school-age children. Her husband's parents lived next door. She said her marriage was good, although her husband suggested she "go see someone" so that she would not be "yelling at everyone all the time." While historically sociable, she rarely talked to her own mother and sisters, much less her friends. A regular churchgoer, she had quit attending because she felt her faith was "weak." Her pastor had always been supportive, but she had not contacted him with her problems because "he wouldn't want to hear about these kinds of issues."

Ms. Smith described herself as having been an outgoing, friendly child. She grew up with her parents and three siblings. She recalled feeling quite upset at age 10–11 when her parents divorced and her mom remarried. Because of fights with other kids at school, she met with a school counselor with whom she felt a bond. Unlike the psychiatrist she had recently consulted, Ms. Smith felt the counselor did not "get into my business" and helped her recover. She said she became quieter as she entered junior high school, with fewer friends and little interest in studying. She married her husband at age 20 and worked in retail sales until the birth of their first child when she was 23 years old.

Ms. Smith had not used alcohol since her first pregnancy and denied any use of illicit substances. She denied past and current use of prescribed medications, other than the brief trial of the antidepressant medication. She reported generally good health.

On mental status examination, Ms. Smith was a casually groomed young woman who was coherent and goal directed. She had difficulty making eye contact with the white middle-aged therapist. She was cooperative but mildly guarded and slow to respond. She needed encouragement to elaborate her thinking. She was periodically tearful and generally appeared sad. She denied psychosis, although she reported occasionally feeling mistrustful of her family. She denied confusion, hallucinations, suicidality, and homicidality. Cognition, insight, and judgment were all considered normal.

Diagnosis

• Major depressive disorder, moderate, with melancholic features

Discussion

Ms. Smith presents with 8–10 months of a persistently depressed mood, anhedonia, poor sleep, diminished appetite with weight loss, anergia, and thoughts of death. She easily meets the requirement of five of nine symptom criteria for a major depression. There is no evidence that the symptoms are caused by a substance or another medical condition. She is distressed and dysfunctional to an extent that warrants clinical attention. She therefore meets criteria for DSM-5 major depressive disorder (MDD). In addition, Ms. Smith has classic melancholic features: she reports loss of pleasure in almost all activities, describes a distinct quality of depressed mood (characterized by profound despondency or despair), is regularly worse in the morning, has had significant weight loss, and is feeling excessive guilt.

Ms. Smith's irritability is prominent. Irritability may be more readily endorsed than sadness, especially by African Americans, among whom psychiatric stigma is high. A complaint of irritability can be part of mania or hypomania, but Ms. Smith lacks other symptoms of mania.

An important depression specifier is whether the MDD is a single episode or recurrent. It is not clear whether Ms. Smith had a major depression after her parents' divorce when she was a child. To clarify, the clinician should explore further those long-ago symptoms. It is interesting that she was referred to a school counselor at that time because of irritability and fights with classmates.

Knowledge of her parents' divorce might have helped teachers recognize that she was in a depression, but it would not have been unusual for her to have been labeled "impulsive and disruptive" rather than a depressed young girl who needed help.

More information about the intervening course is also needed to determine whether Ms. Smith has had sufficiently persistent sad mood (2 years, more days than not) to consider an additional diagnosis of persistent depressive disorder (dysthymia). Persistent major depression is more common among blacks than whites, as is greater severity and disability, despite lower overall prevalence of major depression. Lower use of mental health services by African Americans and delays in seeking treatment may contribute to illness persistence, as may lower rates of antidepressant medication use. Ms. Smith discontinued fluoxetine because it made her tired, but it may have been that she was mistrustful of medication and her prior therapist.

Ms. Smith is wary of mental health professionals. She did not like her previous psychiatrist "getting into [her] business," and she did not make good eye contact with her most recent psychiatrist, who is described as white and middle-aged. Differences in racial, ethnic, and socioeconomic characteristics may affect treatment alliance and adherence, and Ms. Smith's outcome may depend partly on her therapist's ability to tactfully address the culturally based mistrust that is likely to affect Ms. Smith's treatment.

Suggested Readings

Alegría M, Chatterji P, Wells K, et al: Disparity in depression treatment among racial and ethnic minority populations in the United States. Psychiatr Serv 59(11): 1264–1272, 2008

Cooper LA, Roter DL, Carson KA, et al: The associations of clinicians' implicit attitudes about race with medical visit communication and patient ratings of interpersonal care. Am J Public Health 102(5):979–987, 2012

Fava M, Hwang I, Rush AJ, et al: The importance of irritability as a symptom of major depressive disorder: results from the National Comorbidity Survey Replication. Mol Psychiatry 15(8):856–867, 2010

González HM, Croghan T, West B, et al: Antidepressant use in black and white populations in the United States. Psychiatr Serv 59(10):1131–1138, 2008

González HM, Vega WA, Williams DR, et al: Depression care in the United States: too little for too few. Arch Gen Psychiatry 67(1):37–46, 2010

Neighbors HW, Caldwell C, Williams DR, et al: Race, ethnicity, and the use of services for mental disorders: results from the National Survey of American Life. Arch Gen Psychiatry 64(4):485–494, 2007

Williams DR, González HM, Neighbors H, et al: Prevalence and distribution of major depressive disorder in African Americans, Caribbean blacks, and non-Hispanic whites: results from the National Survey of American Life. Arch Gen Psychiatry 64(3):305–315, 2007

Case 6: Feeling Low for Years

Benjamin Brody, M.D.

Diane Taylor, a 35-year-old laboratory technician, was referred to the outpatient psychiatry department of an academic medical center by the employee assistance program (EAP) of her employer, a major pharmaceutical company. Her supervisor had referred Ms. Taylor to the EAP after she had become tearful while being mildly criticized during an otherwise positive annual performance review. Somewhat embarrassed, she told the consulting psychiatrist that she had been "feeling low for years" and that hearing criticism of her work had been "just too much."

A native of western Canada, Ms. Taylor came to the United States to pursue graduate studies in chemistry. She left graduate school before completing her doctorate and began work as a laboratory technician. She felt frustrated with her job, which she saw as a "dead end," yet feared that she lacked the talent to find more satisfying work. As a result, she struggled with guilty feelings that she "hadn't done much" with her life.

Despite her troubles at work, Ms. Taylor felt that she could concentrate without difficulty. She denied ever having active suicidal thoughts, yet sometimes wondered,

"What is the point of life?" When asked, she reported that she occasionally had trouble falling asleep. However, she denied any change in her weight or appetite. Although she occasionally would go out with coworkers, she said that she felt shy and awkward in social situations unless she knew the people well. She did enjoy jogging and the outdoors. Although her romantic relationships tended to "not last long," she felt that her sex drive was normal. She noted that her symptoms waxed and waned but had remained consistent over the past 3 years. She had no symptoms suggestive of mania or hypomania.

Ms. Taylor was an only child. Growing up, she had a close relationship with her father, a pharmacist who owned a drugstore. She described him as a "normal guy who liked to hunt and fish" and liked to take her hiking. Her mother, a nurse, stopped working shortly after giving birth and had seemed emotionally distant and depressed.

Ms. Taylor became depressed for the first time in high school when her father was repeatedly hospitalized after developing leukemia. At that time she was treated with psychotherapy and responded well. She had no other psychiatric or medical history, and her medications were a multivitamin and oral contraceptives. When offered several different treatments, she expressed a preference for a combination of medication and psychotherapy. She started taking citalopram and began a course of supportive psychotherapy. After several months of treatment, she revealed that she had been sexually abused by a family friend during her childhood. It also emerged that she had few women friends and a persistent pattern of dysfunctional and occasionally abusive relationships with men.

Diagnosis

- Persistent depressive disorder (dysthymia)

Discussion

It has long been recognized that depressive illnesses are not always episodic, and a significant minority of patients suffer from chronic forms of depression with varying degrees of severity. Early versions of DSM characterized mild, chronic depression as a personality disorder. In DSM-III, however, the milder form of chronic depression was introduced as an affective illness called dysthymic disorder. That move reflected a growing body of research suggesting that the condition can respond to antidepressant medication, but the move was controversial. Do these patients feel dysphoric *because* of their chronic social dysfunction, occupational difficulties, and morose cognitive styles? Alternatively, does their chronic underlying depression lead to an atrophy of their relationships and interpersonal skills and a selective attentional bias to negative life events?

When first conceptualized in DSM-III, dysthymia was described as being a less severe but more chronic variant of acute major depression. Evidence accumulated, however, that "pure" dysthymia (i.e., persistent mild depression without episodes of major depression) was uncommon. This led to the description of a spectrum of chronic depressions, of which dysthymia was the most mild. Slightly more severe was "double depression," or a major depressive episode superimposed on a baseline dysthymic state. The next most severe involved two or more major depressive episodes bridged by periods of incomplete improvement. Two years of symptoms severe enough to meet full criteria for MDD represented the most severe form. In practice, many patients found it difficult to recall their symptom fluctuations well enough to make these distinctions meaningful. DSM-5 now aggregates contemporary descriptions of these patterns as specifiers under the diagnosis persistent depressive disorder (dysthymia).

Does Ms. Taylor meet the criteria for this DSM-5 diagnosis? She has certainly had chronic symptoms. Despite significant occupational and interpersonal impairment, she endorses psychological but not neurovegetative symptoms of depression, which fall below the threshold for major depression. However, whether that has consistently been the case over the past 2 years is difficult to tell. It is possible, for example, that although Ms. Taylor denied difficulty concentrating at the time of evaluation, her employers may have felt otherwise at times in the past. The DSM-5 criteria allow for the possibility that although she may have slipped into major depression at times, the current diagnosis is still persistent depressive disorder (dysthymia).

The interplay of affective illness and personality also emerges from Ms. Taylor's story. She manifests personality traits (anxiousness, withdrawal, restricted affectivity, intimacy avoidance, and sensitivity to criticism) that shape how she sees the world and can perpetuate her depressive symptoms. Whether or not Ms. Taylor meets criteria for a comorbid avoidant personality disorder, these personality traits are liable to complicate treatment and portend a poor outcome. Alternatively, these dysfunctional personality traits may improve with resolution of her dysthymic symptoms.

Suggested Readings

Blanco C, Okuda M, Markowitz JC, et al: The epidemiology of chronic major depressive disorder and dysthymic disorder: results from the National Epidemiologic Survey on Alcohol and Related Conditions. J Clin Psychiatry 71(12):1645–1656, 2010

Kocsis JH, Frances AJ: A critical discussion of DSM-III dysthymic disorder. Am J Psychiatry 144(12):1534–1542, 1987

Case 7: Mood Swings

Margaret Altemus, M.D.

Emma Wang, a 26-year-old investment banker, referred herself to an outpatient psychiatrist because of "mood swings" that were ruining her relationship with her boyfriend.

She said their latest argument was triggered by his being slightly late for a date. She had yelled at him and then, out of the blue, ended the relationship. She felt despondent afterward, guilty and self-critical. When she called him to make up, he had refused, saying he was tired of her "PMS explosions." She had then cut herself superficially on her left forearm, which she had found to be a reliable method to reduce anxiety since she was a young teenager.

She said these mood swings came out of the blue every month and that they featured tension, argumentativeness, anxiety, sadness, and regret. Sometimes she yelled at her boyfriend, but she also got upset with friends, work, and her family. During the week in which she was "Mr. Hyde," she avoided socializing or talking on the phone; she wouldn't be her "usual fun self," she said, and would alienate her friends. She was able to work when she felt "miserable," but she did have relatively poor energy and concentration. She was also edgy and "self-pitying" and regretful that she had chosen to "waste" her youth working so hard for an uncaring financial institution.

When she was feeling "desperate," she would be determined to seek treatment. Soon after the onset of her period, she would improve dramatically, return to her old self, and not find the time to see a psychiatrist. During the several weeks after her period, she said she felt "fine, terrific, the usual."

She said the mood swings always started 7–10 days before the start of her menstrual period, "like terrible PMS." Her periods were regular. She had premenstrual breast tenderness, bloating, increased appetite, and weight gain. Almost as soon as her period began, she felt "suddenly good." She denied alcohol or illicit substance use and had no history of psychotic, manic, or obsessional symptoms. She denied any suicidal thoughts and any prior suicide attempts and psychiatric hospitalizations. She denied allergies and medical problems. She took one medication, her birth control pill. Her family history was pertinent for a mother with possible depression. Ms. Wang was born in Taiwan and came to the United States at age 14 to attend boarding school. After graduating from an elite business school, she moved in with her older sister.

On mental status examination, Ms. Wang was a fashionably dressed East Asian woman wearing tasteful jewelry and carrying a designer bag. Her hair was slightly askew. She maintained good eye contact and was pleasant and cooperative throughout the interview. Her speech was normal in rate, rhythm, and volume. She described her mood as "generally good," and her affect was full, reactive, and mildly irritable. Her thought process was linear, and she showed no evidence of delusions, obsessions, or hallucinations. She denied suicidal and homicidal ideation. Her insight, judgment, and impulse control were intact, although she noted a history of perimenstrual impairment in these areas.

Diagnosis

• Premenstrual dysphoric disorder

Discussion

Ms. Wang presents with mood swings, irritability, nonsuicidal self-injury (cutting), interpersonal instability, anxiety, sadness, social withdrawal, diminished concentration and energy, and anhedonia. She also describes physical symptoms such as increased appetite, clumsiness, fatigue, and bloating. These symptoms are severe enough to impair her social relationships and her function at work.

This history could fit a number of psychiatric disorders, but Ms. Wang also indicates that these symptoms occur only during a circumscribed time before the onset of her menses. At other times of the month, she is upbeat, energetic, and optimistic. Disappearance of symptoms after onset of menses is key to the diagnosis of DSM-5 premenstrual dysphoric disorder (PMDD).

Ms. Wang reports 7–10 days of symptoms premenstrually, which is on the longer end of the spectrum of symptom duration for PMDD. Some women have symptoms starting at ovulation and lasting for 2 weeks, but a shorter duration of symptoms is more common. Among women with premenstrual symptoms, the most symptomatic days, averaging across all women, are the 4 days preceding and the 2 days following onset of menses.

Ms. Wang's cutting behavior is not typical of PMDD. Impaired impulse control suggests borderline traits in addition to PMDD symptoms. Comorbid disorders do not exclude the diagnosis of PMDD. Many psychiatric disorders have exacerbations during the premenstrual period, but in such cases the patient does not return to her normal self after the menstrual period begins. Ms. Wang suggests that she has "PMS," or premenstrual syndrome, which is a medical condition but not a DSM-5 diagnosis. Criteria for PMS tend to be less rigorous than for PMDD and do not require an affective component.

PMDD is not associated with abnormalities in circulating levels of estrogen or progesterone. Instead, women with PMDD seem to be more sensitive to normal luteal hormone fluctuations. Hormone blood levels are, therefore, not part of the diagnostic evaluation. Although hormonal contraceptives might be expected to help with symptoms, women taking oral contraceptives often continue to have premenstrual mood symptoms (as seen in Ms. Wang).

One component that is crucial in making the PMDD diagnosis is an accurate longitudinal history. Retrospective symptom reports are often inaccurate throughout psychiatry, and that is true for premenstrual symptoms. Validated scales are available for assessing PMDD, such as the Daily Record of Severity of Problems. At this early stage of evaluation, DSM-5 would indicate that Ms.Wang has a provisional diagnosis of PMDD. Only after she has recorded symptoms over two menstrual cycles could she be said to have DSM-5 PMDD.

Suggested Readings

Hartlage SA, Freels S, Gotman N, et al: Criteria for premenstrual dysphoric disorder: secondary analyses of relevant data sets. Arch Gen Psychiatry 69(3): 300–305, 2012

Yonkers KA, O'Brien PM, Eriksson E: Premenstrual syndrome. Lancet 371(9619):1200–1210, 2008

Case 8: Stress, Drugs, and Unhappiness

Edward V. Nunes, M.D.

Frank Young, a 40-year-old business executive, was brought for a psychiatric consultation by his wife. While Mr. Young sat quietly beside her, she reported that a change had come over him during the last 6 months. He was either quiet and withdrawn or uncharacteristically irritable. He had begun to drink alcohol to excess in social situations, sometimes embarrassing her. He often came home late, or not at all, claiming to have been at the office. When away from home, he rarely answered phone calls and text messages. She wondered if he was having an affair. Mr. Young denied seeing anyone else and indicated he had just been having a hard time.

After his wife left the psychiatrist's office, Mr. Young reported a great deal of stress at work over the last year as he tried to deal with industry-wide setbacks and personal financial losses. He said he felt down and depressed most of the time. He reported difficulty sleeping most nights, loss of interest in his wife and children, low energy, and feelings of failure and self-criticism. He had frequent thoughts of wanting to be dead and of suicide, but he denied any suicidal intent or plans.

When asked about the alcohol, he acknowledged that he had been drinking heavily for at least 6 months. When asked about other substances, he asked about therapeutic confidentiality and then acknowledged that he had been using cocaine several times per week for about 9 months. He kept his cocaine use from his wife because he knew she would be judgmental. In the beginning, cocaine put him in a reliably positive, optimistic mood, and he found that he could more successfully churn through large volumes of otherwise tedious and discouraging work. Although his work required some socializing in the evening, he also began to regularly go to bars in the evening just so that he would have a place to comfortably combine cocaine with alcohol. He craved the high from cocaine, went out of his way to obtain it, and spent a lot of time getting high that he would previously have been spending with his family.

When asked to clarify the sequence of work stress, cocaine use, and depression symptoms, he reported that he had felt worried and discouraged about work for a year, but the feelings of depression, loss of interest, irritability, insomnia, and low self-esteem had not begun until about 6 months earlier, 3 months after he had begun to use cocaine regularly. He experienced those depressive symptoms most of the day every day, whether or not he had taken cocaine within the last several days.

Mr. Young denied any previous episodes of depression, other mood or anxiety disorders, or suicide attempts. He drank socially. He had experimented with cannabis and cocaine as a teenager but had never developed a pattern of regular use or impairment until the past year.

Diagnoses

- Cocaine use disorder, moderate severity
- Substance-induced major depressive disorder

Discussion

Mr. Young has significant depression. He meets criteria for cocaine use disorder of at least moderate severity and may also have an alcohol use disorder. He also has significant work stress and appears to be in a tense marriage. The relationships between his mood, his substance use, and his stress are complicated but crucial to the development of an effective treatment strategy.

The first difficulty in evaluating substance use disorders is getting an accurate history about behaviors that are often embarrassing and illegal. Mr. Young was quite forthcoming about his cocaine use, but only after he was specifically asked about alcohol and substance use. Waiting for patients to spontaneously report illicit substance use is more likely to lead to not getting the information. This is problematic given that substance use is widespread and frequently co-occurs with other psychiatric disorders. An empathic, nonjudgmental interviewing style will usually help the patient open up. In other words, asking about alcohol and common drugs of abuse with a matter-of-fact attitude indicates to the patient that his or her answers will not be surprising and will provide information that can improve the treatment. As seen with Mr. Young, family members are often the ones to bring a substance-abusing patient to consultation. They can be important allies in clarifying the symptoms and implementing a treatment plan. Mr. Young needed time alone with the clinician to tell his story, but it was very useful to hear his wife's observations.

A careful exploration of the history can help differentiate between diagnoses that are associated with similar symptoms. Cocaine withdrawal typically causes depressive symptoms, for example, as do a major depression and a substance-induced depression. One important differentiating factor is the temporal relationship between symptoms and the use of the substances.

A primary major depression would be diagnosed if the depression began before the onset of substance abuse or persisted for a substantial period of time beyond cessation of substance use. The amount of time is left to the clinician's judgment, but about 1 month is suggested. Major depression would also be diagnosed if the involved substance is deemed unlikely to cause a depressive syndrome or if the patient had previously experienced recurrent non-substance-induced major depressions. Mr. Young had never had a major depression until after he started abusing cocaine, and there has not been a substantial abstinent period since, so primary major depression cannot be diagnosed.

It is also important to consider the possibility that Mr. Young's symptoms are the direct result of intoxication and/or withdrawal. Intoxication with and withdrawal from cocaine and alcohol can cause depressed mood and sleep disturbance, but symptoms would be expected to resolve within a day or two of the last use. Mr. Young's depression and insomnia persist, regardless of the timing of his last use. In addition, other depressive symptoms such as suicidal ideation are not typically part of intoxication or withdrawal.

Mr. Young, therefore, is diagnosed with a substance-induced depression, which is linked to depressions that appear to have been induced by the ongoing use of a substance and that seem to have taken on a life of their own. If Mr. Young's depression persists after a month of abstinence, his diagnosis would shift to a major depression, although the clinician would likely consider the cocaine to have triggered the depression.

It is useful to identify substance-induced depression. Compared to independent major depressions, substance-induced depression is associated with an increased suicide risk. Furthermore, the additional depression diagnosis reduces the likelihood that someone with a substance use disorder will achieve abstinence. Substance-induced depression should be kept on a patient's list of diagnoses and followed carefully.

Suggested Readings

Compton WM, Thomas YF, Stinson FS, et al: Prevalence, correlates, disability, and comorbidity of DSM-IV drug abuse and dependence in the United States: results from the National Epidemiologic Survey on Alcohol and Related Conditions. Arch Gen Psychiatry 64(5): 566–576, 2007

Hasin D, Liu X, Nunes E, et al: Effects of major depression on remission and relapse of substance dependence. Arch Gen Psychiatry 59(4):375–380, 2002

Hasin DS, Stinson FS, Ogburn E, et al: Prevalence, correlates, disability, and comorbidity of DSM-IV alcohol abuse and dependence in the United States: results from the National Epidemiologic Survey on Alcohol and Related Conditions. Arch Gen Psychiatry 64(7):830–842, 2007

Nunes EV, Liu X, Samet S, et al: Independent versus substance-induced major depressive disorder in substance-dependent patients: observational study of course during follow-up. J Clin Psychiatry 67(10):1561–1567, 2006

Ramsey SE, Kahler CW, Read JP, et al: Discriminating between substance-induced and independent depressive episodes in alcohol dependent patients. J Stud Alcohol 65(5):672–676, 2004

Case 9: Coping With Parkinson's Disease

Thomas W. Meeks, M.D.

George Anderson, a 79-year-old man, was referred to a psychiatrist for an evaluation of depression. For most of the 6 years since his diagnosis with Parkinson's disease (PD), Mr. Anderson had coped well and continued to engage in many of his usual activities.

Three months prior to the referral, however, Mr. Anderson began to decline social invitations from family and friends. He reported that he had withdrawn socially because he had lost pleasure in things that used to excite him, although he denied persistent feelings of sadness or worry. He recognized that he was not his "usual self" and tried, to no avail, to give himself "pep talks." He had worked as a high school science teacher until retirement at age 67, and reported having learned "the power of seeing the glass half full" from his students. He felt frustrated that he could not "snap out of it" for the first time in his life but was hopeful about getting professional help. He denied wishing for death, explaining that although he was not afraid of death, he wanted to enjoy life as long as possible. He added, "God does not give me more than I can handle. I can't ask for a better family, and I have had a full life."

Other new symptoms noted over the prior few months included increasing fatigue, trouble with concentration and memory, unintentional weight loss (7% of his body mass index over 2 months), and restless sleep with initial insomnia.

His wife of 54 years had also noticed that for nearly 2 years, Mr. Anderson had been thrashing his body in the bed halfway through the night, occasionally striking her in his sleep. When he awoke from such an incident, he was coherent and often reported he had been dreaming of swimming or running from something. His wife took over driving shortly after his PD diagnosis, but he was otherwise independent in activities of daily living such as paying bills and managing his medications. His wife described him as "maybe a little more forgetful" over the past few years, but neither of them was concerned about this mild memory loss.

Past medical history included prostate cancer (in remission), glaucoma, and gout. Family psychiatric history was positive only for a granddaughter with autism. He reported no past troublesome substance use and drank a glass of wine two or three times a year. He denied any previous depressive episodes, psychiatric treatment, or psychiatric evaluations.

On mental status examination, Mr. Anderson was pleasant, cooperative, and interpersonally engaging. He had a mild to moderate resting tremor, shuffling gait, hypophonia, and bradykinesia. He occasionally smiled, but his affect was difficult to gauge due to significant masked facies. He reported his mood as "blah." There was no evidence of psychosis.

On cognitive testing, he had some difficulty on the Trail Making Test part B, figure copying, and word-list recall, the latter being helped by category prompts. He scored 25 out of 30 on the Montreal Cognitive Assessment (MCA).

Diagnoses

- Depressive disorder due to another medical condition (Parkinson's disease), with major depressive–like episode
- Rapid eye movement (REM) sleep behavior disorder

Discussion

Although Mr. Anderson denies sad mood, he does have evidence of anhedonia along with five other depressive symptoms (appetite/weight loss, insomnia, fatigue, poor concentration, and psychomotor retardation), all for greater than 2 weeks. These symptoms are distressing to him and are significantly impacting his social functioning. This could indicate major depressive disorder (MDD). However, Mr. Anderson has no personal or family history of depressive disorders, an atypically late age at onset, symptom development during the course of PD, and no identifiable acute life stressor. Clinically significant depression occurs in approximately one of three PD cases. Thus, it is more likely that his depressive symptoms are related to physiological changes in the central nervous system caused by PD.

When depressive symptoms are temporally associated with the onset or progression of another medical condition, and are not explained by delirium, the DSM-5 diagnosis "depressive disorder due to another medical condition" should be considered. This diagnosis is intended for situations in which the direct *physiological* effects of another medical condition (e.g., neurodegeneration in PD) cause depressive symptoms. In other words, this diagnosis is not intended to describe individuals whose symptoms derive from a psychological reaction to illness, which would instead be classified as an adjustment disorder, with depressed mood. These two possible etiologies of depressive symptoms (physiological versus psychological) are somewhat artificially dichotomized and may coexist. There are, however, many cases when the evidence heavily suggests one more than the other. Mr. Anderson's previous resiliency in the face of developing PD and his ongoing positive coping style make the diagnosis of adjustment disorder less likely.

If the criteria for symptom duration and number are met for MDD, the specifier "with major depressive-like episode" should be added to the diagnosis. Because symptoms from a nonpsychiatric medical illness can overlap with depressive symptoms, diagnostic ambiguity may arise. For instance, persons with PD often experience symptoms such as fatigue, psychomotor retardation, sleep disturbance, cognitive impairment, and weight loss independent of depressed mood or anhedonia. However, in Mr. Anderson's case, these symptoms developed or worsened in conjunction with his new-onset anhedonia, which suggests a major depressive–like episode due to another medical condition.

As often occurs in PD, Mr. Anderson has a sleep disturbance consistent with REM sleep behavior disorder. This sleep disorder is characterized by "repeated episodes of arousal during sleep associated with vocalization and/or complex motor behaviors" that may result in "injury to self or the bed partner." Upon awakening, affected persons typically have a clear sensorium and a sense of having "acted out" their dreams. Polysomnography would reveal absence of atonia during REM sleep but would not be required in order to make the diagnosis in the context of a synucleinopathy such as PD. Symptoms typically occur 90 minutes or more into sleep and more often in the second half of the night, when REM sleep is more common. Although Mr. Anderson's history is consistent with REM sleep behavior disorder, his new initial insomnia is not explained by this diagnosis and is more consistent with depression.

Cognitive changes, particularly impairments of visuospatial, executive, and memory retrieval functions, often occur in PD. Mr. Anderson's MCA results are typical of such cognitive changes, but his new-onset subjective difficulty with concentration is more likely secondary to depression. His cognitive problems are mild and not overtly impairing; he does not meet criteria for an independent neurocognitive disorder, although prospective monitoring of cognition would be wise, given that 25%–30% of persons with PD develop dementia.

In addition to meeting criteria for two DSM-5 disorders, Mr. Anderson displays evidence of resilience, wisdom, and other signs of psychological health. He demonstrates positive coping skills (e.g., cognitive reframing, use of social supports), long-term healthy relationships, spirituality, gratitude, optimism, and developmentally appropriate ego integrity. He also exhibits a healthy, nonmorbid perspective about personal mortality. Unfortunately, even individuals with few risk factors for depression and with evidence of lifelong healthy psychological functioning are not immune to the neuropsychiatric effects of certain medical conditions.

Suggested Readings

Aarsland D, Zaccai J, Brayne C: A systematic review of prevalence studies of dementia in Parkinson's disease. Mov Disord 20(10):1255–1263, 2005

Boeve BF: Idiopathic REM sleep behaviour disorder in the development of Parkinson's disease. Lancet Neurol 12(5):469–482, 2013

Gallagher DA, Schrag A: Psychosis, apathy, depression and anxiety in Parkinson's disease. Neurobiol Dis 46(3):581–589, 2012

Jeste DV, Ardelt M, Blazer D, et al: Expert consensus on characteristics of wisdom: a Delphi method study. Gerontologist 50(5):668–680, 2010

Jeste DV, Savla GN, Thompson WK, et al: Association between older age and more successful aging: critical role of resilience and depression. Am J Psychiatry 170(2):188–196, 2013

Case 10: Situational Mood Swings

Joseph F. Goldberg, M.D.

Helena Bates was a 27-year-old single administrative assistant who presented for a psychiatric evaluation and treatment for depression. She had recently begun an intensive outpatient program after a first lifetime hospitalization for an impulsive overdose following the breakup of a 2-year relationship. She said she had been feeling increasingly sad and hopeless for 1–2 months in anticipation of the breakup. About a month prior to admission, she began seeing a new psychotherapist who told her she had "borderline traits" and "situational mood swings."

During these 4–8 weeks, Ms. Bates's mood had been moderately depressed throughout the day most days, with no diurnal variation and intact mood reactivity. She had recently gained about 10 pounds from "overeating comfort food and junk." She denied prominent irritability or argumentativeness. She described her self-esteem as "none" and had found it hard to feel motivation or to concentrate on routine tasks. By contrast, sometimes she would have "bursts" of nonstop thinking about her estranged boyfriend and devising ways to "get him back," alternating with "grieving his loss." She described times of being flooded with strategies to regain his interest (including purchasing a full-page newspaper "open letter" to him) and recently found herself awake until 5:00 or 6:00 A.M. journaling or calling friends in the middle of the night "for support." She would then "trudge through the day" without fatigue after only 2–3 hours of sleep. These symptoms began prior to her hospitalization. She denied drug or alcohol misuse and self-injurious behavior. Until this particular breakup, she denied a history of particularly intense or chaotic relationships, as well as a history of suicidal thoughts or gestures. Indeed, Ms. Bates seemed horrified by her own overdose, which occurred in the context of a depression.

Previously, Ms. Bates had seen a counselor in high school for "moodiness" and poor grades. She became "depressed" in college. At that time, she began escitalopram and psychotherapy, but improved quickly and stopped both after a few weeks. While in the hospital following her suicide attempt, she started taking vilazodone and quetiapine at bedtime "for sleep."

Ms. Bates was the youngest of three children who grew up in a middle-class suburban home. She attended public school and a state college as "mostly a B student" and hoped to someday go to law school. She described herself as having been a "quiet, anxious" child and "not a troublemaker." Her older brother abused multiple substances, although Ms. Bates said she herself had never used illicit substances. Her younger sister was treated for "panic attacks and depression," and Ms. Bates knew of several aunts and cousins whom she thought were "depressed."

On examination, Ms. Bates was a pleasant, well-related, casually but appropriately dressed, moderately overweight woman, appearing her stated age, who made good eye contact. Her speech was somewhat rapid and verbose but interruptible and non-pressured. She had no abnormal motor movements, but she gestured dramatically and with excessive animation. Her mood was depressed, and her affect was tense and dysphoric but with full range and normal responsivity. Ms. Bates's thought processes were somewhat circumstantial but generally coherent, linear, and logical. Her thought content was notable for passive thoughts that she might be better off dead, but without intent or plan; she had no delusions, hallucinations, or homicidal thoughts. Her higher integrative functioning was grossly intact, as were her insight and judgment.

Diagnosis

•   Major depressive disorder with mixed features

Discussion

Ms. Bates meets DSM-5 criteria for a major depressive episode, manifesting pervasive depressed mood with at least five associated features (suicidal thoughts, poor concentration, low self-esteem, hyperphagia, and psychomotor agitation). She also describes several symptoms consistent with mania or hypomania: a decreased need for sleep with nocturnal hyperactivity and no consequent next-day fatigue, probable racing thoughts, and rapid, verbose speech (as noted on interview). Although the examiner deemed Ms. Bates's insight and judgment globally intact at the time of the interview, some of her recent thoughts (e.g., posting an open letter in a newspaper) and actions (calling friends in the middle of the night) suggest impaired judgment involving behaviors with the potential for painful consequences.

Although Ms. Bates does have some manic symptoms, she does not meet DSM-5 requirements for a diagnosis of mania or hypomania. She would be said to have subsyndromal hypomania along with the syndromal depression. This combination qualifies her for a new diagnosis in DSM-5: major depressive disorder with mixed features. Previously, "mixed features" applied only to bipolar I disorder, whereas the term can now modify major depression and both bipolar I and bipolar II disorders.

The DSM-5 construct of unipolar depression with mixed features reflects observations that many unipolar depressed patients display subthreshold signs of hypomania. DSM-5 "disallows" counting four potential manic/hypomanic symptoms, because they can also reflect major depression—namely, insomnia (as opposed to decreased need for sleep), distractibility, indecisiveness, and irritability. DSM-5 identifies "abnormally and persistently increased activity or energy" as a mandatory criterion for diagnosing bipolar II hypomania, but this feature is not necessary to define unipolar depression with mixed features. In the present case, if Ms. Bates had irritable mood in addition to her racing thoughts, rapid speech, and decreased need for sleep, she would meet DSM-5 criteria for bipolar II hypomania, and the mixed features specifier would then apply by virtue of her concomitant depressive symptoms.

The DSM-5 mixed features specifier requires that symptoms of the opposite polarity (in this case, mania/hypomania) be present "almost every day during the episode." This latter criterion means that if Ms. Bates's manic/hypomanic symptoms had been present for fewer than 4 days (the minimum duration criterion for diagnosing bipolar II hypomania), her subthreshold hypomania symptoms would not count toward either a "mixed" or a "manic/hypomanic" designation and her diagnosis would simply be unipolar major depression. Some authors have criticized DSM-5's stringency of discounting subthreshold hypomania symptoms if they involve only *two* manic/hypomanic symptoms or if they fail to persist for the full duration of an episode, because such presentations (referred to in the literature as "depressive mixed states") have been observed when as few as two mania/hypomania symptoms coexist with syndromal unipolar depression for as few as 2–4 days, and represent a construct that more closely resembles bipolar than unipolar disorder in family history, age at onset, and suicide risk.

One might speculate that Ms. Bates's psychomotor activation and subthreshold hypomania could have arisen as a consequence of the recent introduction of the selective serotonin reuptake inhibitor (SSRI) vilazodone. However, in this case, the history indicates that her hypomanic symptoms predated her hospitalization and SSRI introduction; it would be important for the examiner to determine that this chronology is accurate (which would suggest that her mixed symptoms are not iatrogenic), because the mixed features specifier requires that symptoms be "not attributable to the physiological effects of a substance." Note that this qualifying statement is in contrast to the DSM-5 criteria for a manic/mixed/hypomanic episode, insofar as the emergence of mania/hypomania symptoms associated with recent antidepressant exposure is now classified as a bipolar disorder (similar to the viewpoint in DSM-III-R) and no longer as a substance-induced mood disorder (as in DSM-IV-TR).

Major depression patients with subthreshold hypomania have about a 25% chance of eventually developing a full mania or hypomania. Therefore, although not all major depression patients who display subthreshold mixed features will develop syndromal mania or hypomania, such patients warrant particularly careful evaluation, treatment, and longitudinal monitoring.

Ms. Bates's symptoms of impulsivity and hyperactivity may have contributed to her acute presentation being wrongly identified as borderline personality disorder. Her longitudinal history does not support a pattern of symptoms suggestive of borderline personality disorder, and her suicide attempt and affective instability are readily accounted for by a current full affective syndrome.

Suggested Readings

Angst J, Cui L, Swendsen J, et al: Major depressive disorder with subthreshold bipolarity in the National Comorbidity Survey Replication. Am J Psychiatry 167(10):1194–1201, 2010

Fiedorowicz JG, Endicott J, Leon AC, et al: Subthreshold hypomanic symptoms in progression from unipolar major depression to bipolar disorder. Arch Gen Psychiatry 168(1):40–48, 2011

Goldberg JF, Perlis RH, Ghaemi SN, et al: Adjunctive antidepressant use and symptomatic recovery among bipolar depressed patients with concomitant manic symptoms: findings from the STEP-BD. Am J Psychiatry 164(9):1348–1355, 2007

Sato T, Bottlender R, Schröter A, et al: Frequency of manic symptoms during a depressive epi-
      sode and unipolar 'depressive mixed state' as bipolar spectrum. Acta Psychiatr Scand
      107(4):268–274, 2003

Case 11: Floundering

Peter D. Kramer, M.D.

Ian Campbell was a 32-year-old man who presented for psychiatric consultation
because he was floundering at work. When he failed to make progress on a simple
project, his boss expressed concern. Mr. Campbell offered that he had been distracted
by problems at home. More seemed wrong, the boss suggested. Mr. Campbell phoned
his internist, who sent him to a neurologist, who referred Mr. Campbell for psychiatric evaluation.

Mr. Campbell had encountered this problem, difficulty concentrating, before. In college, after his father died of a chronic illness, Mr. Campbell had been unable to study
and had taken time off. Twice at his prior job, he experienced episodes lasting months
in which he had difficulty making decisions. One of these intervals followed a romantic setback.

Mr. Campbell's mother and sister had been diagnosed with major depression and
treated successfully with medication. A maternal uncle had committed suicide.

The current impairment's onset accompanied the breakdown of Mr. Campbell's
marriage of 6 years. Two months earlier, his wife had filed for divorce, announcing that
she would live in the distant city her work had taken her to. Mr. Campbell had expected to feel relief; he said his wife had been hostile throughout the marriage. He had
begun to entertain fond thoughts of a coworker. Nevertheless, he felt "flat"—unable to
imagine a future.

Closer questioning revealed that Mr. Campbell's problems went beyond impaired
cognition. He described apathy and diminished energy. Jazz was a passion, but he no
longer attended recitals—although impaired concentration probably played a role as
well. Listening, the psychiatrist noted probable retardation of speech. Mr. Campbell
said that his employer had mentioned that Mr. Campbell was moving in slow motion.
The problems were worse in the mornings. In the evenings, Mr. Campbell noticed a
spark of energy. He put on music and reviewed reports ignored during the workday.

Mr. Campbell declined to characterize himself as sad. He was pleased that the marriage was ending. But the psychiatrist was struck by her own affect in Mr. Campbell's
presence; she felt glum, pessimistic, even weepy.

She questioned Mr. Campbell at length about depressed mood, changed sleep and
appetite, feelings of guilt or worthlessness, and thoughts of death. None of these at-
tributions, he said, applied. Nor had he had indicators of disorders that can be confused with depression. He was not dysthymic; between episodes of impairment, he
felt and functioned well.

The psychiatrist decided that the problem at hand was close enough to depression
to warrant treatment. Factors that influenced her decision included the partial syn-

dromal presentation, diurnal variation, periodic recurrence, lack of future orientation, and her own empathic experience. She proposed psychotherapy centered on Mr. Campbell's decompensation in the face of loss. He insisted that he did not see the impending divorce in that light. The two agreed on brief psychotherapy supplemented by antidepressants. Within weeks, Mr. Campbell was functioning at full capacity. During the treatment, the psychiatrist was unable to elicit evidence of depressive symptoms beyond those noted in the initial history. All the same, she was convinced that the impaired concentration was a sign and symptom of something very much like major depression.

Diagnosis

• Other specified depressive disorder (depressive episode with insufficient symptoms)

Discussion

The operational definition of major depression, which reached official standing in the third edition of DSM, is one of the great inventions in modern medicine. The approach has catalyzed productive research in fields ranging from cell biology to social psychiatry. Most of what is known about mood disorder, from the abnormalities it represents in the brain to the harm it does in lives, arises from the delineation of depression out of the inchoate domain of neurosis and psychosis.

That said, the definition is arbitrary. Historians have traced the DSM criteria to a 1957 *Journal of the American Medical Association* article whose lead author, a Boston psychiatrist, Walter Cassidy, had tried to systematize the study of a condition similar to today's major depression. For diagnosis, Cassidy required that patients have six of 10 symptoms from a list that included slow thinking, poor appetite, loss of concentration, and others that remain current. Later asked how he chose six, Cassidy said, "It sounded about right."

Operational approaches to depression, from DSM to the Hamilton Rating Scale for Depression, are attempts to create reliability in the face of an inherently ill-defined phenomenon—that is, clinicians' working diagnoses. Psychiatrists identified depressed patients using prevailing methods—sometimes with attention to their own empathic resonance with the patient; the symptom- and severity-based definitions translated the impressionistic into reproducible form.

Depression, however, has no known natural boundary. Behavioral geneticists find the DSM criteria arbitrary. Number, severity, and duration of symptoms each represent a continuum of disability. Patients who suffer four severe symptoms of depression for 2 weeks tend to do badly down the road. Five moderately disabling symptoms for 10 days confer a poor prognosis. Five mild symptoms, if they persist, predict substantial risk.

In this case, Mr. Campbell appears not to have had the five of nine criteria necessary for a diagnosis of major depression, but he would likely qualify for a DSM-5 diagnosis of other specified depressive disorder (depressive episode with insufficient symptoms). It is important to recognize that depression's harm—suffering, future full episodes, work and social problems, suicide—is only slightly less in people who narrowly miss full criteria. In one analysis, later major depression was as common in those who reported three or four symptoms as in those who reported five. Estimates of heritability are similar, too; "minor" depression in one sibling predicts full depression in an identical twin. One form of other specified depressive disorder appears especially dangerous: recurrent brief depression is associated with high rates of attempted suicide.

The DSM-5 categories unspecified and other specified depressive disorders acknowledge an important clinical reality: effectively, the near penumbra of depression *is* depression. Low-level episodes can appear as precursors of major depression and as sequelae, even in the absence of dysthymia; on its own, low-level depression represents suffering and confers risk.

Mr. Campbell's doctor will want to take his complaints seriously. Mr. Campbell may have entered a "depressive episode with insufficient symptoms," but the insufficiency relates to the symptom count for a major depressive episode, not to the level of illness needed to trigger clinical concern. Especially when peripheral factors—such as, in this case, the diurnal variation typical of classic depression—suggest mood disorder, the clinician will suspect that effectively the condition *is* depression and will approach the situation with the corresponding urgency and thoroughness.

Suggested Readings

Cassidy WL, Flanagan NB, Spellman M, et al: Clinical observations in manic-depressive disease: a quantitative study of one hundred manic-depressive patients and fifty medically sick controls. J Am Med Assoc 164(14):1535–1546, 1957

Havens L: A Safe Place: Laying the Groundwork of Psychotherapy. Cambridge, MA, Harvard University Press, 1989

Kendler KS, Gardner CO Jr: Boundaries of major depression: an evaluation of DSM-IV criteria. Am J Psychiatry 155(2): 172–177, 1998

Kendler KS, Muñoz RA, Murphy G: The development of the Feighner criteria: a historical perspective. Am J Psychiatry 167(2):134–142, 2010

Kramer P: Against Depression. New York, Viking, 2005

Pezawas L, Angst J, Gamma A, et al: Recurrent brief depression—past and future. Prog Neuropsychopharmacol Biol Psychiatry 27(1):75–83, 2003

Case 12: Insomnia and Physical Complaints

Russell F. Lim, M.D.

Ka Fang, a 59-year-old widowed Hmong woman, was referred to a mental health clinic after she recurrently complained to her primary care physician of fatigue, chronic back pain, and insomnia. Over the preceding 11 months, the internist had prescribed clonazepam for sleep and Vicodin for pain. Her sleep had improved and her pain decreased, but she continued to feel tired all day. At that point, the internist referred her for the psychiatric evaluation.

Ka had immigrated to the United States from Thailand a few years earlier. Natives of Laos, she and her family had spent almost two decades in a Thai refugee camp following the Vietnam War. Her family had resettled in the Sacramento area with the assistance of a local church group.

When questioned using a Hmong interpreter, Ka denied depressed mood. When asked if she enjoyed things, she said that she felt privileged to be in America and had no right to complain. She said she felt she was not doing enough to help her family. She was embarrassed by her fatigue because she did not "do anything all day." She denied any intention to harm herself.

She said she was very proud of all her children, especially her son, who had been an excellent student in Thailand and spoke good English. Nevertheless, her son, his wife, and their two young children followed many of the cultural practices that they had followed in Laos and Thailand, and often prepared Hmong food for dinner. He and his wife had bought a small farm outside Sacramento and were doing well, cultivating Asian vegetables. Her son had employed her two daughters on the farm until both had moved back to live in the Hmong community in Sacramento.

Ka indicated that the transition to California had gone better than she had expected. The biggest disappointments for her had been her husband's unexpected death from a heart attack 1 year earlier and the fact that most of her extended family had remained in Thailand.

On mental status examination, the patient was short and heavyset. She wore a floral short-sleeve blouse, black polyester slacks, black flip-flops, and no makeup. She had white strings tied around her wrists. Her eyes were generally downcast, but she seemed alert. She appeared sad and constricted but denied feeling depressed. Her speech was slow and careful. She denied all hallucinations, suicidality, and homicidality. Cognitive testing revealed normal attention and concentration but little formal education; she appeared to be functionally illiterate. Her insight into her illness appeared limited.

When asked about the strings around her wrists, Ka explained that she had recently sought out a Hmong shaman, who had organized several soul-calling ceremonies to reunite with distant relatives.

Diagnosis

- Other specified depressive disorder (depressive episode with insufficient symptoms)

Discussion

Ka presents for an evaluation of psychiatric contributions to her fatigue, insomnia, and pain. She endorses symptoms of insomnia, feelings of worthlessness, and fatigue, but she denies a depressed mood, anhedonia, agitation, weight loss, poor concentration, or thoughts of suicide. She fulfills only three of nine DSM-5 major depression criteria; five are needed to make the diagnosis.

Ka reports a number of pertinent cultural issues. She lives in a Hmong-speaking household with her son and his family on their farm outside of Sacramento. They raise vegetables, their apparent occupation when they lived in Laos and Thailand. In Hmong culture, the young married couple generally lives with the family of the husband, making the mother-in-law especially prominent. Although Ka expresses her appreciation for her situation, she may still feel marginalized and lonely, especially in the context of her husband's recent death and her daughters having moved back to the

Hmong community in Sacramento. Being functionally illiterate—not uncommon in societies in which limited educational resources are primarily channeled to boys—Ka is not able to avail herself of tools to maintain connections, such as e-mail and newspapers. Her feelings of isolation are likely connected to the strings that the interviewer noticed on her wrists. Shamanistic soul-calling ceremonies are intended to reunite families, and she may be especially in need given her distance from her daughters, her Southeast Asian home, her Hmong culture, her extended family, and her ancestors.

In assessing whether Ka has a mood disorder, it is useful to know that there is no word in the Hmong language for depression. Like many people from other cultures, Ka describes somatic symptoms such as insomnia, anergia, and bodily aches to express depressed feelings. These probably are not adequate to meet symptomatic criteria for a DSM-5 major depressive disorder, and, by report, her symptoms have not yet persisted for the 2 years required for dysthymic disorder. It would be useful to get collateral information from one of her children, who might be able to provide information that could solidify the diagnosis. As it stands, she best fits the DSM-5 diagnosis other specified depressive disorder (depressive episode with insufficient symptoms).

Suggested Readings

Culhane-Pera KA, Vawter DE, Xiong P, et al: Healing by Heart: Clinical and Ethical Case Stories of Hmong Families and Western Providers. Nashville, TN, Vanderbilt University Press, 2003

Lim RF: Clinical Manual of Cultural Psychiatry. Washington, DC, American Psychiatric Publishing, 2006

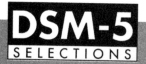

Depressive Disorders

DSM-5® Self-Exam Questions

1. How does DSM-5 differ from DSM-IV in its classification of mood disorders?

   A. There is no difference between the two editions.
   B. DSM-IV separated mood disorders into different sections; DSM-5 consolidates mood disorders into one section.
   C. DSM-IV included all mood disorders in a single section; DSM-5 places depressive and bipolar mood disorders in separate sections.
   D. DSM-IV placed mood and anxiety disorders in separate sections; DSM-5 consolidates mood and anxiety disorders within a single section.
   E. DSM-IV placed mood disorders with psychotic features in the same section as other mood disorders; DSM-5 places mood disorders with psychosis in a separate section.

2. How does DSM-5 differ from DSM-IV in its classification of premenstrual dysphoric disorder (PMDD)?

   A. PMDD was in the Appendix in DSM-IV and remains in this location in DSM-5.
   B. PMDD was not included in DSM-IV but is in the Appendix of DSM-5.
   C. PMDD is no longer considered a valid psychiatric diagnosis.
   D. PMDD is included in the "Depressive Disorders" chapter of DSM-5 but was not included in the "Mood Disorders" chapter of DSM-IV.
   E. PMDD is included in DSM-5 but the name of the diagnosis has been changed.

3. What DSM-5 diagnostic provision is made for depressive symptoms following the death of a loved one?

   A. Depressive symptoms lasting less than 2 months after the loss of a loved one are excluded from receiving a diagnosis of major depressive episode.
   B. To qualify for a diagnosis of major depressive episode, the depression must start no less than 12 weeks following the loss.
   C. To qualify for a diagnosis of major depressive episode, the depressive symptoms in such individuals must include suicidal ideation.
   D. Depressive symptoms following the loss of a loved one are not excluded from receiving a major depressive episode diagnosis if the symptoms otherwise fulfill the diagnostic criteria.

E. Depressive symptoms following the loss of a loved one are excluded from receiving a major depressive episode diagnosis; however, a proposed diagnostic category for postbereavement depression is included in "Conditions for Further Study" (DSM-5 Appendix) pending further research.

4. Which of the following statements about how grief differs from a major depressive episode (MDE) is *false?*

   A. In grief the predominant affect is feelings of emptiness and loss, while in MDE it is persistent depressed mood and the inability to anticipate happiness or pleasure.
   B. The pain of grief may be accompanied by positive emotions and humor that are uncharacteristic of the pervasive unhappiness and misery characteristic of MDE.
   C. The thought content associated with grief generally features a preoccupation with thoughts and memories of the deceased, rather than the self-critical or pessimistic ruminations seen in MDE.
   D. In grief, feelings of worthlessness and self-loathing are common; in MDE, self-esteem is generally preserved.
   E. If a bereaved individual thinks about death and dying, such thoughts are generally focused on the deceased and possibly about "joining" the deceased, whereas in MDE such thoughts are focused on ending one's own life because of feeling worthless, undeserving of life, or unable to cope with the pain of depression.

5. How do individuals with substance/medication-induced depressive disorder differ from individuals with major depressive disorder who do not have a substance use disorder?

   A. They are more likely to be female.
   B. They are more likely to have graduate school education.
   C. They are more likely to be male.
   D. They are more likely to be white.
   E. They are less likely to report suicidal thoughts/attempts.

6. A 50-year-old man presents with persistently depressed mood for several weeks that interferes with his ability to work. He has insomnia and fatigue, feels guilty, has thoughts he would be better off dead, and has thought about how he could die without anyone knowing it was a suicide. His wife informs you that he requests sex several times a day and that she thinks he may be going to "massage parlors" regularly, both of which are changes from his typical behavior. He has told her he has ideas for a "better Internet," and he has invested thousands of dollars in software programs that he cannot use. She notes that he complains of fatigue but sleeps only 1 or 2 hours each night and seems to have tremendous energy during the day. Which diagnosis best fits this patient?

A. Manic episode.
B. Hypomanic episode.
C. Major depressive episode.
D. Major depressive episode, with mixed features.
E. Major depressive episode, with atypical features.

7. A 45-year-old man with classic features of schizophrenia has always experienced co-occurring symptoms of depression—including feeling "down in the dumps," having a poor appetite, feeling hopeless, and suffering from insomnia—during his episodes of active psychosis. These depressive symptoms occurred only during his psychotic episodes and only during the 2-year period when the patient was experiencing active symptoms of schizophrenia. After his psychotic episodes were successfully controlled by medication, no further symptoms of depression were present. The patient has never met full criteria for major depressive disorder at any time. What is the appropriate DSM-5 diagnosis?

A. Schizophrenia.
B. Schizoaffective disorder.
C. Persistent depressive disorder (dysthymia).
D. Schizophrenia and persistent depressive disorder (dysthymia).
E. Unspecified schizophrenia spectrum and other psychotic disorder.

8. What are the new depressive disorder diagnoses in DSM-5?

A. Subsyndromal depressive disorder, premenstrual dysphoric disorder, and mixed anxiety and depressive disorder.
B. Disruptive mood dysregulation disorder, premenstrual dysphoric disorder, and persistent depressive disorder (dysthymia).
C. Disruptive mood dysregulation disorder, premenstrual dysphoric disorder, and subsyndromal depressive disorder.
D. Disruptive mood dysregulation disorder, postmenopausal dysphoric disorder, and persistent depressive disorder (dysthymia).
E. Mixed anxiety and depressive disorder, bereavement-induced major depressive disorder, and postmenopausal dysphoric disorder.

9. A depressed patient reports that he experiences no pleasure from his normally enjoyable activities. Which of the following additional symptoms would be required for this patient to qualify for a diagnosis of major depressive disorder with melancholic features?

A. Despondency, depression that is worse in the morning, and inability to fall asleep.
B. Depression that is worse in the evening, psychomotor agitation, and significant weight loss.
C. Inappropriate guilt, depression that is worse in the morning, and early-morning awakening.

D. Significant weight gain, depression that is worse in the evening, and excessive guilt.

E. Despondency, significant weight gain, and psychomotor retardation.

10. A 39-year-old woman reports that she became quite depressed in the winter last year when her company closed for the season, but she felt completely normal in the spring. She recalls experiencing several other episodes of depression over the past 5 years (for which she cannot identify a seasonal pattern) that would have met criteria for major depressive disorder. Which of the following correctly summarizes this patient's eligibility for a diagnosis of "major depressive disorder, with seasonal pattern"?

A. She does *not* qualify for this diagnosis: the episode must start in the fall, and the patient must have no episodes that do not have a seasonal pattern.

B. She *does* qualify for this diagnosis: the single episode described started in the winter and ended in the spring.

C. She does *not* qualify for this diagnosis: the patient must have had two episodes with a seasonal relationship in the past 2 years and no nonseasonal episodes during that period.

D. She *does* qualify for this diagnosis: the symptoms described are related to psychosocial stressors.

E. She *does* qualify for this diagnosis: the symptoms are not related to bipolar I or bipolar II disorder.

11. Which of the following statements about the prevalence of major depressive disorder in the United States is *true?*

A. The 12-month prevalence is 17%.

B. Females and males have equal prevalence at all ages.

C. Females have increased prevalence at all ages.

D. The prevalence in 18- to 29-year-olds is three times higher than that in 60-year-olds.

E. The prevalence in 60-year-olds is three times higher than that in 18- to 29-year-olds.

12. Which of the following statements about the heritability of major depressive disorder (MDD) is *true?*

A. Nearly 100% of people with genetic liability can be accounted for by the personality trait of dogmatism.

B. The heritability is approximately 40%, and the personality trait of neuroticism accounts for a substantial portion of this genetic liability.

C. Less than 10% of people with genetic liability can be accounted for by the personality trait of perfectionism.

D. Nearly 50% of people with genetic liability can be accounted for by the personality trait of aggressiveness.

E. The heritability of MDD depends on whether the individual's mother or father had MDD.

13. Which of the following statements about diagnostic markers for major depressive disorder (MDD) is *true?*

    A. No laboratory test has demonstrated sufficient sensitivity and specificity to be used as a diagnostic tool for MDD.
    B. Several diagnostic laboratory tests exist, but no commercial enterprise will offer them to the public.
    C. Diagnostic laboratory tests have been withheld for fear that people testing positive for MDD may attempt suicide.
    D. Tests that exist are adequate diagnostically but are not covered by health insurance.
    E. Only functional magnetic resonance imaging (fMRI) provides absolute diagnostic reliability for MDD.

14. Which of the following statements about gender differences in suicide risk and suicide rates in major depressive disorder (MDD) is *true?*

    A. The risk of suicide attempts and completions is higher for women.
    B. The risk of suicide attempts and completions is higher for men.
    C. The risk of suicide attempts and completions is equal for men and women.
    D. The disparity in suicide rate by gender is much greater in individuals with MDD than in the general population.
    E. The risk of suicide attempts is higher for women, but the risk of suicide completions is lower.

15. A 12-year-old boy begins to have new episodes of temper outbursts that are out of proportion to the situation. Which of the following is *not* a diagnostic possibility for this patient?

    A. Disruptive mood dysregulation disorder.
    B. Bipolar disorder.
    C. Oppositional defiant disorder.
    D. Conduct disorder.
    E. Attention-deficit/hyperactivity disorder.

16. Which of the following features distinguishes disruptive mood dysregulation disorder (DMDD) from bipolar disorder in children?

    A. Age at onset.
    B. Gender of the child.
    C. Irritability.
    D. Chronicity.
    E. Severity.

17. Children with disruptive mood dysregulation disorder are most likely to develop which of the following disorders in adulthood?

    A. Bipolar I disorder.
    B. Schizophrenia.
    C. Bipolar II disorder.
    D. Borderline personality disorder.
    E. Unipolar depressive disorders.

18. An irritable 8-year-old child has a history of temper outbursts both at home and at school. What characteristic mood feature must be also present to qualify him for a diagnosis of disruptive mood dysregulation disorder?

    A. The child's mood between outbursts is typically euthymic.
    B. The child's mood between outbursts is typically hypomanic.
    C. The child's mood between outbursts is typically depressed.
    D. The child's mood between outbursts is typically irritable or angry.
    E. The mood symptoms and temper outbursts must not have persisted for more than 6 months.

19. Children with disruptive mood dysregulation disorder (DMDD) often meet criteria for what additional DSM-5 diagnosis?

    A. Pediatric bipolar disorder.
    B. Oppositional defiant disorder.
    C. Schizophrenia.
    D. Intermittent explosive disorder.
    E. Major depressive disorder.

20. The diagnostic criteria for disruptive mood dysregulation disorder (DMDD) state that the diagnosis should not be made for the first time before age 6 years or after 18 years (Criterion G). Which of the following statements best describes the rationale for this age range restriction?

    A. Validity of the diagnosis has been established only in the age group 7–18 years.
    B. The restriction represents an attempt to differentiate DMDD from bipolar disorder.
    C. The restriction is based on existing genetic data.
    D. The restriction represents an attempt to differentiate DMDD from intermittent explosive disorder.
    E. The restriction represents an attempt to differentiate DMDD from autism spectrum disorder.

21. A 9-year-old boy is brought in for evaluation because of explosive outbursts when he is frustrated with schoolwork. The parents report that their son is well behaved and pleasant at other times. Which diagnosis best fits this clinical picture?

A. Disruptive mood dysregulation disorder.
B. Pediatric bipolar disorder.
C. Intermittent explosive disorder.
D. Major depressive disorder.
E. Persistent depressive disorder (dysthymia).

22. A 14-year-old boy describes himself as feeling "down" all of the time for the past year. He remembers feeling better while he was at camp for 4 weeks during the summer; however, the depressed mood returned when he came home. He reports poor concentration, feelings of hopelessness, and low self-esteem but denies suicidal ideation or changes in his appetite or sleep. What is the most likely diagnosis?

    A. Major depressive disorder.
    B. Disruptive mood dysregulation disorder.
    C. Depressive episodes with short-duration hypomania.
    D. Persistent depressive disorder (dysthymia), with early onset.
    E. Schizoaffective disorder.

23. A 30-year-old woman reports 2 years of persistently depressed mood, accompanied by loss of pleasure in all activities, ruminations that she would be better off dead, feelings of guilt about "bad things" she has done, and thoughts about quitting work because of her inability to make decisions. Although she has never been treated for depression, she feels so distressed at times that she wonders if she should be hospitalized. She experiences an increased need for sleep but still feels fatigued during the day. Her overeating has led to a 12-kg weight gain. She denies drug or alcohol use, and her medical workup is completely normal, including laboratory tests for vitamins. The consultation was prompted by her worsened mood for the past several weeks. What is the most appropriate diagnosis?

    A. Major depressive disorder (MDD).
    B. Persistent depressive disorder (dysthymia), with persistent major depressive episode.
    C. Cyclothymia.
    D. Bipolar II disorder.
    E. MDD, with melancholic features.

24. A 45-year-old woman with multiple sclerosis was treated with interferon beta-1a a year ago, which resolved her physical symptoms. She now presents with depressed mood (experienced daily for the past several months), middle insomnia (of recent onset), poor appetite, trouble concentrating, and lack of interest in sex. Although she has no physical symptoms, she is frequently absent from work. She denies any active plans to commit suicide but admits that she often thinks about it, as her mood has worsened. What is the most likely diagnosis?

    A. Major depressive disorder.
    B. Persistent depressive disorder (dysthymia).
    C. Depressive disorder due to another medical condition.

    D. Substance/medication-induced depressive disorder.

    E. Persistent depressive disorder (dysthymia) and multiple sclerosis.

25. An 18-year-old college student, recently arrived in the United States from Beijing, complains to her gynecologist of irritability, problems with her roommates, increased appetite, feeling bloated, and feeling depressed for 3–4 days prior to the onset of menses. She reports that these symptoms have been present since she reached menarche at age 12 (although she has never kept a mood log). The gynecologist calls you for a consultation about the correct diagnosis, because she is as yet unfamiliar with the new DSM-5 diagnostic criteria. What is your response?

    A. The patient has premenstrual syndrome because she does not meet criteria for premenstrual dysphoric disorder.

    B. The patient would qualify for a provisional diagnosis of premenstrual dysphoric disorder; however, the diagnosis does not exist in DSM-5.

    C. The patient would qualify for a provisional diagnosis of premenstrual dysphoric disorder.

    D. The patient would qualify for a provisional diagnosis of premenstrual dysphoric disorder if the diagnosis had been validated in Asian women.

    E. The patient has no DSM-5 diagnosis.

26. What is the appropriate method of confirming a diagnosis of premenstrual dysphoric disorder?

    A. Laboratory tests.

    B. Family history.

    C. Neuropsychological testing.

    D. Two or more months of prospective symptom ratings on validated scales.

    E. One month of scoring high on the Daily Rating of Severity of Problems or 1 month of scoring high on the Visual Analogue Scales for Premenstrual Mood Symptoms.

27. A 29-year-old woman complains of sad mood every month in anticipation of her very painful menses. The pain begins with the start of her flow and continues for several days. She does not experience pain during other times of the month. She has tried a variety of treatments, none of which have given her relief. What is the appropriate diagnosis?

    A. Premenstrual dysphoric disorder.

    B. Premenstrual syndrome.

    C. Dysmenorrhea.

    D. Factitious disorder.

    E. Persistent depressive disorder (dysthymia).

28. Which of the following symptoms must be present for a woman to meet criteria for premenstrual dysphoric disorder?

    A. Marked affective lability.

    B. Decreased interest in usual activities.

    C. Physical symptoms such as breast tenderness.

    D. Marked change in appetite.

    E. A sense of feeling overwhelmed or out of control.

29. A 23-year-old woman reports that during every menstrual cycle she experiences breast swelling, bloating, hypersomnia, an increased craving for sweets, poor concentration, and a feeling that she cannot handle her normal responsibilities. She notes that she also feels somewhat more sensitive emotionally and may become tearful when hearing a sad story. She takes no oral medication but does use a drospirenone/ethinyl estradiol patch. What diagnosis best fits this clinical picture?

    A. Premenstrual dysphoric disorder (PMDD).

    B. Dysthymia.

    C. Dysmenorrhea.

    D. Premenstrual syndrome.

    E. Substance/medication-induced depressive disorder.

30. A 31-year-old woman with no history of mood symptoms reports that she experiences distressing mood lability and irritability starting about 4 days before the onset of menses. She feels "on edge," cannot concentrate, has little enjoyment from any of her activities, and experiences bloating and swelling of her breasts. The patient reports that these symptoms started 6 months ago when she began taking oral contraceptives for the first time. If she stops the oral contraceptives and her symptoms remit, what would the diagnosis be?

    A. Premenstrual dysphoric disorder.

    B. Dysthymia.

    C. Major depressive episode.

    D. Substance/medication-induced depressive disorder.

    E. Premenstrual syndrome.

31. A 45-year-old man is admitted to the hospital with profound hypothyroidism. He is depressed but does not meet full criteria for major depressive disorder (MDD), the diagnosis given to him by his internist. The patient has no prior history of a mood disorder, and all of the depressive symptoms are temporally related to the hypothyroidism. Based on this information, you determine that a change in diagnosis—to depressive disorder due to another medical condition—is warranted, as well as a specifier to indicate that full criteria for MDD are not met. How would the full diagnosis be recorded?

    A. Hypothyroidism would be coded on Axis III in DSM-5.

    B. There is no special coding procedure in DSM-5.

    C. Hypothyroidism would be recorded as the name of the "other medical condition" in the DSM-5 diagnosis.

    D. Medical disorders are not coded as part of a mental disorder diagnosis in DSM-5.

    E. A revision to DSM-5 is planned to deal with this issue.

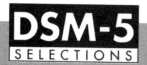

Depressive Disorders

DSM-5® Self-Exam Answer Guide

1. How does DSM-5 differ from DSM-IV in its classification of mood disorders?

   A. There is no difference between the two editions.
   B. DSM-IV separated mood disorders into different sections; DSM-5 consolidates mood disorders into one section.
   C. DSM-IV included all mood disorders in a single section; DSM-5 places depressive and bipolar mood disorders in separate sections.
   D. DSM-IV placed mood and anxiety disorders in separate sections; DSM-5 consolidates mood and anxiety disorders within a single section.
   E. DSM-IV placed mood disorders with psychotic features in the same section as other mood disorders; DSM-5 places mood disorders with psychosis in a separate section.

   Correct Answer: C. DSM-IV included all mood disorders in a single section; DSM-5 places depressive and bipolar mood disorders in separate sections.

   Explanation: Unlike DSM-IV, DSM-5 separates depressive disorders from bipolar and related disorders, and several new disorders have been added. "With psychotic features" is a specifier for bipolar and depressive disorders; there is no separate diagnostic section for mood disorders with psychotic symptoms.

   1—chapter intro (p. 155)

2. How does DSM-5 differ from DSM-IV in its classification of premenstrual dysphoric disorder (PMDD)?

   A. PMDD was in the Appendix in DSM-IV and remains in this location in DSM-5.
   B. PMDD was not included in DSM-IV but is in the Appendix of DSM-5.
   C. PMDD is no longer considered a valid psychiatric diagnosis.
   D. PMDD is included in the "Depressive Disorders" chapter of DSM-5 but was not included in the "Mood Disorders" chapter of DSM-IV.
   E. PMDD is included in DSM-5 but the name of the diagnosis has been changed.

   Correct Answer: D. PMDD is included in the "Depressive Disorders" chapter of DSM-5 but was not included in the "Mood Disorders" chapter of DSM-IV.

Explanation: After careful scientific review of the evidence, PMDD has been moved from Appendix B ("Criteria Sets and Axes Provided for Further Study") of DSM-IV to Section II of DSM-5. Almost 20 years of additional research on this condition has confirmed a specific and treatment-responsive form of depressive disorder that begins sometime following ovulation and remits within a few days of menses and has a marked impact on functioning.

2—chapter intro (p. 155)

3. What DSM-5 diagnostic provision is made for depressive symptoms following the death of a loved one?

    A. Depressive symptoms lasting less than 2 months after the loss of a loved one are excluded from receiving a diagnosis of major depressive episode.
    B. To qualify for a diagnosis of major depressive episode, the depression must start no less than 12 weeks following the loss.
    C. To qualify for a diagnosis of major depressive episode, the depressive symptoms in such individuals must include suicidal ideation.
    D. Depressive symptoms following the loss of a loved one are not excluded from receiving a major depressive episode diagnosis if the symptoms otherwise fulfill the diagnostic criteria.
    E. Depressive symptoms following the loss of a loved one are excluded from receiving a major depressive episode diagnosis; however, a proposed diagnostic category for postbereavement depression is included in "Conditions for Further Study" (DSM-5 Appendix) pending further research.

Correct Answer: D. Depressive symptoms following the loss of a loved one are not excluded from receiving a major depressive episode diagnosis if the symptoms otherwise fulfill the diagnostic criteria.

Explanation: In DSM-IV, there was an exclusion criterion for a major depressive episode that was applied to depressive symptoms lasting less than 2 months following the death of a loved one (i.e., the bereavement exclusion). This exclusion is omitted in DSM-5 for several reasons, including the recognition that bereavement is a severe psychosocial stressor that can precipitate a major depressive episode in a vulnerable individual, generally beginning soon after the loss, and can add an additional risk of suffering, feelings of worthlessness, suicidal ideation, poorer medical health, and worse interpersonal and work functioning. It was critical to remove the implication that bereavement typically lasts only 2 months, when both physicians and grief counselors recognize that the duration is more commonly 1–2 years. A detailed footnote has replaced the more simplistic DSM-IV exclusion to aid clinicians in making the critical distinction between the symptoms characteristic of bereavement and those of a major depressive disorder.

3—Appendix / Highlights of Changes From DSM-IV to DSM-5 / Depressive Disorders (pp. 810–811)

4. Which of the following statements about how grief differs from a major depressive episode (MDE) is *false?*

   A. In grief the predominant affect is feelings of emptiness and loss, while in MDE it is persistent depressed mood and the inability to anticipate happiness or pleasure.
   B. The pain of grief may be accompanied by positive emotions and humor that are uncharacteristic of the pervasive unhappiness and misery characteristic of MDE.
   C. The thought content associated with grief generally features a preoccupation with thoughts and memories of the deceased, rather than the self-critical or pessimistic ruminations seen in MDE.
   D. In grief, feelings of worthlessness and self-loathing are common; in MDE, self-esteem is generally preserved.
   E. If a bereaved individual thinks about death and dying, such thoughts are generally focused on the deceased and possibly about "joining" the deceased, whereas in MDE such thoughts are focused on ending one's own life because of feeling worthless, undeserving of life, or unable to cope with the pain of depression.

Correct Answer: D. In grief, feelings of worthlessness and self-loathing are common; in MDE, self-esteem is generally preserved.

Explanation: In distinguishing grief from an MDE, it is useful to consider that in grief the predominant affect is feelings of emptiness and loss, while in MDE it is persistent depressed mood and the inability to anticipate happiness or pleasure. The dysphoria in grief is likely to decrease in intensity over days to weeks and occurs in waves, the so-called pangs of grief. These waves tend to be associated with thoughts or reminders of the deceased. The depressed mood of MDE is more persistent and not tied to specific thoughts or preoccupations. The pain of grief may be accompanied by positive emotions and humor that are uncharacteristic of the pervasive unhappiness and misery characteristic of MDE. The thought content associated with grief generally features a preoccupation with thoughts and memories of the deceased, rather than the self-critical or pessimistic ruminations seen in MDE. In grief, self-esteem is generally preserved, whereas in MDE feelings of worthlessness and self-loathing are common. If self-derogatory ideation is present in grief, it typically involves perceived failings vis-à-vis the deceased (e.g., not visiting frequently enough, not telling the deceased how much he or she was loved). If a bereaved individual thinks about death and dying, such thoughts are generally focused on the deceased and possibly about "joining" the deceased, whereas in MDE such thoughts are focused on ending one's own life because of feeling worthless, undeserving of life, or unable to cope with the pain of depression.

4—Major Depressive Episode / diagnostic criteria (pp. 160–162)

5. How do individuals with substance/medication-induced depressive disorder differ from individuals with major depressive disorder who do not have a substance use disorder?

   A. They are more likely to be female.
   B. They are more likely to have graduate school education.
   C. They are more likely to be male.
   D. They are more likely to be white.
   E. They are less likely to report suicidal thoughts/attempts.

   Correct Answer: C. They are more likely to be male.

   Explanation: In a representative U.S. adult population, compared with individuals with major depressive disorder who did not have a substance use disorder, individuals with substance-induced depressive disorder were more likely to be male, to be black, to have at most a high school diploma, to lack insurance, and to have lower family income. They were also more likely to report higher family history of substance use disorders and antisocial behavior, higher 12-month history of stressful life events, a greater number of DSM-IV major depressive disorder criteria, and feelings of worthlessness, insomnia/hypersomnia, and thoughts of death and suicide attempts.

   5—Substance/Medication-Induced Depressive Disorder / Risk and Prognostic Factors (Course modifiers) (p. 179)

6. A 50-year-old man presents with persistently depressed mood for several weeks that interferes with his ability to work. He has insomnia and fatigue, feels guilty, has thoughts he would be better off dead, and has thought about how he could die without anyone knowing it was a suicide. His wife informs you that he requests sex several times a day and that she thinks he may be going to "massage parlors" regularly, both of which are changes from his typical behavior. He has told her he has ideas for a "better Internet," and he has invested thousands of dollars in software programs that he cannot use. She notes that he complains of fatigue but sleeps only 1 or 2 hours each night and seems to have tremendous energy during the day. Which diagnosis best fits this patient?

   A. Manic episode.
   B. Hypomanic episode.
   C. Major depressive episode.
   D. Major depressive episode, with mixed features.
   E. Major depressive episode, with atypical features.

   Correct Answer: D. Major depressive episode, with mixed features.

   Explanation: The specifier "with mixed features" now denotes the coexistence of at least three manic symptoms insufficient to satisfy criteria for a manic episode, within a major depressive episode. This change is based on findings from studies of family history and diagnostic stability showing that the presence of mixed features in an episode of major depressive disorder increases the likelihood that the illness exists in a bipolar spectrum. This likelihood was judged insufficient to assign such individuals a diagnosis of bipolar disorder. The presence of a full manic syndrome within a depressive episode will continue to be an exclusion criterion for a depressive disorder diagnosis, and individuals with this pattern will be considered to have a manic episode.

6—Specifiers for Depressive Disorders / With mixed features (pp. 184–185)

7. A 45-year-old man with classic features of schizophrenia has always experienced co-occurring symptoms of depression—including feeling "down in the dumps," having a poor appetite, feeling hopeless, and suffering from insomnia—during his episodes of active psychosis. These depressive symptoms occurred only during his psychotic episodes and only during the 2-year period when the patient was experiencing active symptoms of schizophrenia. After his psychotic episodes were successfully controlled by medication, no further symptoms of depression were present. The patient has never met full criteria for major depressive disorder at any time. What is the appropriate DSM-5 diagnosis?

    A. Schizophrenia.
    B. Schizoaffective disorder.
    C. Persistent depressive disorder (dysthymia).
    D. Schizophrenia and persistent depressive disorder (dysthymia).
    E. Unspecified schizophrenia spectrum and other psychotic disorder.

Correct Answer: A. Schizophrenia.

Explanation: Depressive symptoms are a common associated feature of chronic psychotic disorders (e.g., schizoaffective disorder, schizophrenia, delusional disorder). A separate diagnosis of persistent depressive disorder is not made if the symptoms occur only during the course of the psychotic disorder (including residual phases).

7—Persistent Depressive Disorder (Dysthymia) / Differential Diagnosis (pp. 170–171)

8. What are the new depressive disorder diagnoses in DSM-5?

    A. Subsyndromal depressive disorder, premenstrual dysphoric disorder, and mixed anxiety and depressive disorder.
    B. Disruptive mood dysregulation disorder, premenstrual dysphoric disorder, and persistent depressive disorder (dysthymia).
    C. Disruptive mood dysregulation disorder, premenstrual dysphoric disorder, and subsyndromal depressive disorder.
    D. Disruptive mood dysregulation disorder, postmenopausal dysphoric disorder, and persistent depressive disorder (dysthymia).
    E. Mixed anxiety and depressive disorder, bereavement-induced major depressive disorder, and postmenopausal dysphoric disorder.

Correct Answer: B. Disruptive mood dysregulation disorder, premenstrual dysphoric disorder, and persistent depressive disorder (dysthymia).

Explanation: Several new diagnoses appear in the DSM-5 "Depressive Disorders" chapter. After careful scientific review of the evidence, premenstrual dysphoric disorder (PMDD) has been moved from Appendix B ("Criteria Sets and Axes Provided for Further Study") of DSM-IV to Section II of DSM-5. Almost 20 years of additional research on this condition has confirmed a specific and treatment-responsive form of depressive disorder that begins sometime following ovulation and remits within a few days of menses and has a marked impact on functioning.

   In order to address concerns about the potential for the overdiagnosis of and treatment for bipolar disorder in children, a new diagnosis, disruptive mood dysregulation disorder (DMDD), referring to the presentation of children with persistent irritability and frequent episodes of extreme behavioral dyscontrol, is added to the depressive disorders for children up to 12 years of age. Its placement in this chapter reflects the finding that children with this symptom pattern typically develop unipolar depressive disorders or anxiety disorders, rather than bipolar disorders, as they mature into adolescence and adulthood.

   A more chronic form of depression, persistent depressive disorder (dysthymia), can be diagnosed when the mood disturbance continues for at least 2 years in adults or 1 year in children. This diagnosis, new in DSM-5, includes the DSM-IV diagnostic categories of chronic major depression and dysthymia.

8—chapter intro (p. 155)

9. A depressed patient reports that he experiences no pleasure from his normally enjoyable activities. Which of the following additional symptoms would be required for this patient to qualify for a diagnosis of major depressive disorder with melancholic features?

    A. Despondency, depression that is worse in the morning, and inability to fall asleep.
    B. Depression that is worse in the evening, psychomotor agitation, and significant weight loss.
    C. Inappropriate guilt, depression that is worse in the morning, and early morning awakening.
    D. Significant weight gain, depression that is worse in the evening, and excessive guilt.
    E. Despondency, significant weight gain, and psychomotor retardation.

Correct Answer: C. Inappropriate guilt, depression that is worse in the morning, and early morning awakening.

Explanation: Two criteria must be met to qualify for the specifier "with melancholic features" for major depressive disorder. Criterion A specifies that one of

the following must be present during the most severe period of the current episode: 1) loss of pleasure in all, or almost all, activities; 2) lack of reactivity to
usually pleasurable stimuli (does not feel much better, even temporarily, when
something good happens). Criterion B specifies that three (or more) of the following must be present: 1) a distinct quality of depressed mood characterized
by profound despondency, despair, and/or moroseness or by so-called empty
mood; 2) depression that is regularly worse in the morning; 3) early-morning
awakening (i.e., at least 2 hours before usual awakening); 4) marked psychomotor agitation or retardation; 5) significant anorexia or weight loss; 6) excessive or inappropriate guilt. The specifier "with melancholic features" can be
applied to the current (or, if the full criteria are not currently met for major depressive episode, to the most recent) major depressive episode in major depressive disorder or in bipolar I or II disorder only if it is the most recent type of
mood episode.

9—Specifiers for Depressive Disorders / With melancholic features (p. 185)

10. A 39-year-old woman reports that she became quite depressed in the winter
    last year when her company closed for the season, but she felt completely nor-
    mal in the spring. She recalls experiencing several other episodes of depression
    over the past 5 years (for which she cannot identify a seasonal pattern) that
    would have met criteria for major depressive disorder. Which of the following
    correctly summarizes this patient's eligibility for a diagnosis of "major depres-
    sive disorder, with seasonal pattern"?

    A. She does *not* qualify for this diagnosis: the episode must start in the fall, and
       the patient must have no episodes that do not have a seasonal pattern.
    B. She *does* qualify for this diagnosis: the single episode described started in
       the winter and ended in the spring.
    C. She does *not* qualify for this diagnosis: the patient must have had two epi-
       sodes with a seasonal relationship in the past 2 years and no nonseasonal
       episodes during that period.
    D. She *does* qualify for this diagnosis: the symptoms described are related to
       psychosocial stressors.
    E. She *does* qualify for this diagnosis: the symptoms are not related to bipolar I
       or bipolar II disorder.

**Correct Answer: C. She does *not* qualify for this diagnosis: the patient must
have had two episodes with a seasonal relationship in the past 2 years and no
nonseasonal episodes during that period.**

Explanation: The "with seasonal pattern" specifier requires a regular temporal
relationship between the onset of major depressive episodes (MDEs) in major
depressive disorder or in bipolar I or bipolar II disorder and a particular time
of the year (e.g., in the fall or winter). The diagnosis excludes cases in which
there is an obvious effect of seasonal-related psychosocial stressors (e.g., regu-

larly being unemployed every winter). Full remissions (or a change from major depression to mania or hypomania) also occur at a characteristic time of the year (e.g., depression disappears in the spring). In the past 2 years, two MDEs must have occurred that demonstrate the temporal seasonal relationships defined above, and no nonseasonal MDEs must have occurred during that same period. Seasonal MDEs must substantially outnumber the nonseasonal MDEs that may have occurred over the individual's lifetime. The specifier "with seasonal pattern" can be applied to the pattern of MDEs in bipolar I disorder, bipolar II disorder, or major depressive disorder, recurrent.

10—Specifiers for Depressive Disorders / With seasonal pattern (pp. 187–188)

11. Which of the following statements about the prevalence of major depressive disorder in the United States is *true?*

    A. The 12-month prevalence is 17%.
    B. Females and males have equal prevalence at all ages.
    C. Females have increased prevalence at all ages.
    D. The prevalence in 18- to 29-year-olds is three times higher than that in 60-year-olds.
    E. The prevalence in 60-year-olds is three times higher than that in 18- to 29-year-olds.

Correct Answer: D. The prevalence in 18- to 29-year-olds is three times higher than that in 60-year-olds.

Explanation: The 12-month prevalence of major depressive disorder in the United States is 7%, with marked differences by age group such that the prevalence in 18- to 29-year-old individuals is threefold higher than the prevalence in individuals age 60 years or older. Females experience 1.5- to 3-fold higher rates than males beginning in early adolescence.

11—Major Depressive Disorder / Prevalence (p. 165)

12. Which of the following statements about the heritability of major depressive disorder (MDD) is *true?*

    A. Nearly 100% of people with genetic liability can be accounted for by the personality trait of dogmatism.
    B. The heritability is approximately 40%, and the personality trait of neuroticism accounts for a substantial portion of this genetic liability.
    C. Less than 10% of people with genetic liability can be accounted for by the personality trait of perfectionism.
    D. Nearly 50% of people with genetic liability can be accounted for by the personality trait of aggressiveness.
    E. The heritability of MDD depends on whether the individual's mother or father had MDD.

Correct Answer: B. The heritability is approximately 40%, and the personality trait of neuroticism accounts for a substantial portion of this genetic liability.

Explanation: First-degree family members of individuals with major depressive disorder have a risk of major depressive disorder two- to fourfold higher than that of the general population. Relative risks appear to be higher for early onset and recurrent forms. Heritability is approximately 40%, and the personality trait neuroticism accounts for a substantial portion of this genetic liability. Neuroticism (negative affectivity) is a well-established risk factor for the onset of major depressive disorder, and high levels appear to render individuals more likely to develop depressive episodes in response to stressful life events.

12—Major Depressive Disorder / Risk and Prognostic Factors (p. 166)

13. Which of the following statements about diagnostic markers for major depressive disorder (MDD) is *true?*

    A. No laboratory test has demonstrated sufficient sensitivity and specificity to be used as a diagnostic tool for MDD.
    B. Several diagnostic laboratory tests exist, but no commercial enterprise will offer them to the public.
    C. Diagnostic laboratory tests have been withheld for fear that people testing positive for MDD may attempt suicide.
    D. Tests that exist are adequate diagnostically but are not covered by health insurance.
    E. Only functional magnetic resonance imaging (fMRI) provides absolute diagnostic reliability for MDD.

Correct Answer: A. No laboratory test has demonstrated sufficient sensitivity and specificity to be used as a diagnostic tool for MDD.

Explanation: Although an extensive literature exists describing neuroanatomical, neuroendocrinological, and neurophysiological correlates of MDD, no laboratory test has yielded results of sufficient sensitivity and specificity to be used as a diagnostic tool for this disorder. Until recently, hypothalamic-pituitary-adrenal axis hyperactivity had been the most extensively investigated abnormality associated with major depressive episodes, and it appears to be associated with melancholia, psychotic features, and risks for eventual suicide. Molecular studies have also implicated peripheral factors, including genetic variants in neurotrophic factors and pro-inflammatory cytokines. Additionally, fMRI studies provide evidence for functional abnormalities in specific neural systems supporting emotion processing, reward seeking, and emotion regulation in adults with major depression.

13—Major Depressive Disorder / Associated Features Supporting Diagnosis (pp. 164–165)

14. Which of the following statements about gender differences in suicide risk and suicide rates in major depressive disorder (MDD) is *true?*

A. The risk of suicide attempts and completions is higher for women.
B. The risk of suicide attempts and completions is higher for men.
C. The risk of suicide attempts and completions is equal for men and women.
D. The disparity in suicide rate by gender is much greater in individuals with MDD than in the general population.
E. The risk of suicide attempts is higher for women, but the risk of suicide completions is lower.

Correct Answer: E. The risk of suicide attempts is higher for women, but the risk of suicide completions is lower.

Explanation: In women, the risk of suicide attempts is higher, and the risk of suicide completions is lower. The disparity in suicide rate by gender is not as great among those with depressive disorders as it is in the population as a whole.

14—Major Depressive Disorder / Gender-Related Diagnostic Issues (p. 167)

15. A 12-year-old boy begins to have new episodes of temper outbursts that are out of proportion to the situation. Which of the following is *not* a diagnostic possibility for this patient?

A. Disruptive mood dysregulation disorder.
B. Bipolar disorder.
C. Oppositional defiant disorder.
D. Conduct disorder.
E. Attention-deficit/hyperactivity disorder.

Correct Answer: A. Disruptive mood dysregulation disorder.

Explanation: Criteria G and H of disruptive mood dysregulation disorder state that the chronological age at onset is at least 6 years (or equivalent developmental level) and the onset is before 10 years.

15—Disruptive Mood Dysregulation Disorder / diagnostic criteria (p. 156)

16. Which of the following features distinguishes disruptive mood dysregulation disorder (DMDD) from bipolar disorder in children?

A. Age at onset.
B. Gender of the child.
C. Irritability.
D. Chronicity.
E. Severity.

Correct Answer: D. Chronicity.

Explanation: The core feature of DMDD is chronic, severe, persistent irritability. This severe irritability has two prominent clinical manifestations, the first of which is frequent temper outbursts. These outbursts typically occur in response to frustration and can be verbal or behavioral (the latter in the form of aggression against property, self, or others).

The clinical presentation of DMDD must be carefully distinguished from presentations of other, related conditions, particularly pediatric bipolar disorder. DMDD was added to DSM-5 to address the considerable concern about the appropriate classification and treatment of children who present with chronic, persistent irritability relative to children who present with classic (i.e., episodic) bipolar disorder.

In DSM-5, the term *bipolar disorder* is explicitly reserved for episodic presentations of bipolar symptoms. DSM-IV did not include a diagnosis designed to capture youths whose hallmark symptoms consisted of very severe, nonepisodic irritability, whereas DSM-5, with the inclusion of DMDD, provides a distinct category for such presentations.

16—Disruptive Mood Dysregulation Disorder / Diagnostic Features (pp. 156–157)

17. Children with disruptive mood dysregulation disorder are most likely to develop which of the following disorders in adulthood?

    A. Bipolar I disorder.
    B. Schizophrenia.
    C. Bipolar II disorder.
    D. Borderline personality disorder.
    E. Unipolar depressive disorders.

Correct Answer: E. Unipolar depressive disorders.

Explanation: Approximately half of children with severe, chronic irritability will have a presentation that continues to meet criteria for the condition 1 year later. Rates of conversion from severe, nonepisodic irritability to bipolar disorder are very low. Instead, children with chronic irritability are at risk to develop unipolar depressive and/or anxiety disorders in adulthood.

17—Disruptive Mood Dysregulation Disorder / Development and Course (p. 157)

18. An irritable 8-year-old child has a history of temper outbursts both at home and at school. What characteristic mood feature must be also present to qualify him for a diagnosis of disruptive mood dysregulation disorder?

    A. The child's mood between outbursts is typically euthymic.
    B. The child's mood between outbursts is typically hypomanic.
    C. The child's mood between outbursts is typically depressed.

D. The child's mood between outbursts is typically irritable or angry.

E. The mood symptoms and temper outbursts must not have persisted for more than 6 months.

Correct Answer: D. The child's mood between outbursts is typically irritable or angry.

Explanation: Criterion D of disruptive mood dysregulation disorder requires that the child's mood between temper outbursts be persistently irritable or angry most of the day, nearly every day, and observable by others (e.g., parents, teachers, peers).

18—Disruptive Mood Dysregulation Disorder / diagnostic criteria (p. 156)

19. Children with disruptive mood dysregulation disorder (DMDD) often meet criteria for what additional DSM-5 diagnosis?

A. Pediatric bipolar disorder.
B. Oppositional defiant disorder.
C. Schizophrenia.
D. Intermittent explosive disorder.
E. Major depressive disorder.

Correct Answer: B. Oppositional defiant disorder.

Explanation: Because chronically irritable children and adolescents typically present with complex histories, the diagnosis of DMDD must be made while considering the presence or absence of multiple other conditions. The differential diagnosis of DMDD from both bipolar disorder and oppositional defiant disorder requires careful consideration. DMDD differs from bipolar disorder in that the former is chronic, whereas the latter is episodic. DMDD differs from oppositional defiant disorder in that very severe irritability is required in the former but not the latter. For this reason, while most children who meet criteria for DMDD will also meet criteria for oppositional defiant disorder, the reverse is not the case.

19—Disruptive Mood Dysregulation Disorder / Differential Diagnosis (pp. 158–160)

20. The diagnostic criteria for disruptive mood dysregulation disorder (DMDD) state that the diagnosis should not be made for the first time before age 6 years or after 18 years (Criterion G). Which of the following statements best describes the rationale for this age range restriction?

A. Validity of the diagnosis has been established only in the age group 7–18 years.

B. The restriction represents an attempt to differentiate DMDD from bipolar disorder.

    C. The restriction is based on existing genetic data.

    D. The restriction represents an attempt to differentiate DMDD from intermittent explosive disorder.

    E. The restriction represents an attempt to differentiate DMDD from autism spectrum disorder.

Correct Answer: A. Validity of the diagnosis has been established only in the age group 7–18 years.

Explanation: By definition, the onset of DMDD (by history or observation) must be before age 10 years (Criterion H), and the diagnosis should not be applied to children with a developmental age of less than 6 years. It is unknown whether the condition presents only in this age-delimited fashion. Because the symptoms of DMDD are likely to change as children mature, use of the diagnosis should be restricted to age groups similar to those in which validity has been established (7–18 years). Approximately half of children with severe, chronic irritability will have a presentation that continues to meet criteria for the condition 1 year later. Rates of conversion from severe, nonepisodic irritability to bipolar disorder are very low. Instead, children with chronic irritability are at risk to develop unipolar depressive and/or anxiety disorders in adulthood.

20—Disruptive Mood Dysregulation Disorder / Development and Course (p. 157)

21. A 9-year-old boy is brought in for evaluation because of explosive outbursts when he is frustrated with schoolwork. The parents report that their son is well behaved and pleasant at other times. Which diagnosis best fits this clinical picture?

    A. Disruptive mood dysregulation disorder.

    B. Pediatric bipolar disorder.

    C. Intermittent explosive disorder.

    D. Major depressive disorder.

    E. Persistent depressive disorder (dysthymia).

Correct Answer: C. Intermittent explosive disorder.

Explanation: Children with intermittent explosive disorder present with instances of severe temper outbursts much like those in children with disruptive mood dysregulation disorder. However, unlike children with disruptive mood dysregulation disorder, children with intermittent explosive disorder do not exhibit persistent disruption in mood between outbursts. Thus, the two diagnoses are mutually exclusive and cannot be made in the same child. For children with outbursts and intercurrent, persistent irritability, the diagnosis of disruptive mood dysregulation disorder should be made. For children with outbursts but no such irritability, the diagnosis of intermittent explosive disorder should be made.

21—Disruptive Mood Dysregulation Disorder / Differential Diagnosis (pp. 158–160)

22. A 14-year-old boy describes himself as feeling "down" all of the time for the past year. He remembers feeling better while he was at camp for 4 weeks during the summer; however, the depressed mood returned when he came home. He reports poor concentration, feelings of hopelessness, and low self-esteem but denies suicidal ideation or changes in his appetite or sleep. What is the most likely diagnosis?

    A. Major depressive disorder.
    B. Disruptive mood dysregulation disorder.
    C. Depressive episodes with short-duration hypomania.
    D. Persistent depressive disorder (dysthymia), with early onset.
    E. Schizoaffective disorder.

    Correct Answer: D. Persistent depressive disorder (dysthymia), with early onset.

    Explanation: The essential feature of persistent depressive disorder (dysthymia) is a depressed mood that occurs for most of the day, for more days than not, for at least 2 years, or at least 1 year for children and adolescents (Criterion A). This disorder represents a consolidation of DSM-IV-defined chronic major depressive disorder and dysthymic disorder. Major depression may precede persistent depressive disorder, and major depressive episodes may occur during persistent depressive disorder. Individuals whose symptoms meet major depressive disorder criteria for 2 years should be given a diagnosis of persistent depressive disorder as well as major depressive disorder.

    Individuals with persistent depressive disorder describe their mood as sad or "down in the dumps." During periods of depressed mood, at least two of the six symptoms from Criterion B are present. Because these symptoms have become a part of the individual's day-to-day experience, particularly in the case of early onset (e.g., "I've always been this way"), they may not be reported unless the individual is directly prompted. During the 2-year period (1 year for children or adolescents), any symptom-free intervals last no longer than 2 months (Criterion C).

    22—Persistent Depressive Disorder (Dysthymia) / Diagnostic Features (pp. 169–170)

23. A 30-year-old woman reports 2 years of persistently depressed mood, accompanied by loss of pleasure in all activities, ruminations that she would be better off dead, feelings of guilt about "bad things" she has done, and thoughts about quitting work because of her inability to make decisions. Although she has never been treated for depression, she feels so distressed at times that she wonders if she should be hospitalized. She experiences an increased need for sleep but still feels fatigued during the day. Her overeating has led to a 12-kg weight gain. She denies drug or alcohol use, and her medical workup is completely normal, including laboratory tests for vitamins. The consultation was prompted by her worsened mood for the past several weeks. What is the most appropriate diagnosis?

A. Major depressive disorder (MDD).

B. Persistent depressive disorder (dysthymia), with persistent major depressive episode.

C. Cyclothymia.

D. Bipolar II disorder.

E. MDD, with melancholic features.

Correct Answer: B. Persistent depressive disorder (dysthymia), with persistent major depressive episode.

Explanation: The essential feature of persistent depressive disorder (dysthymia) is a depressed mood that occurs for most of the day, for more days than not, for at least 2 years. This disorder represents a consolidation of DSM-IV-defined chronic major depressive disorder and dysthymic disorder. Major depression may precede persistent depressive disorder, and major depressive episodes may occur during persistent depressive disorder. Individuals whose symptoms meet major depressive disorder criteria for 2 years should be given a diagnosis of persistent depressive disorder as well as major depressive disorder.

If there is a depressed mood plus two or more symptoms meeting criteria for a persistent depressive episode for 2 years or more, then the diagnosis of persistent depressive disorder is made. The diagnosis depends on the 2-year duration, which distinguishes it from episodes of depression that do not last 2 years. If the symptom criteria are sufficient for a diagnosis of a major depressive episode at any time during this period, then the diagnosis of major depression should be noted, but it is coded not as a separate diagnosis but rather as a specifier with the diagnosis of persistent depressive disorder. If the individual's symptoms currently meet full criteria for a major depressive episode, then the specifier "with intermittent major depressive episodes, with current episode" would be applied. If—as in the patient described in the above vignette—the major depressive episode has persisted for at least a 2-year duration and remains present, then the specifier "with persistent major depressive episode" is used. When full major depressive episode criteria are not currently met but there has been at least one previous episode of major depression in the context of at least 2 years of persistent depressive symptoms, then the specifier "with intermittent major depressive episodes, without current episode" is used. If the individual has not experienced an episode of major depression in the past 2 years, then the specifier "with pure dysthymic syndrome" is used.

23—Persistent Depressive Disorder (Dysthymia) / diagnostic criteria (pp. 168–169); Diagnostic Features (pp. 169–170); Differential Diagnosis (Major depressive disorder) (pp. 170–171)

24. A 45-year-old woman with multiple sclerosis was treated with interferon beta-1a a year ago, which resolved her physical symptoms. She now presents with depressed mood (experienced daily for the past several months), middle insomnia (of recent onset), poor appetite, trouble concentrating, and lack of interest in sex.

Although she has no physical symptoms, she is frequently absent from work. She denies any active plans to commit suicide but admits that she often thinks about it, as her mood has worsened. What is the most likely diagnosis?

A. Major depressive disorder.
B. Persistent depressive disorder (dysthymia).
C. Depressive disorder due to another medical condition.
D. Substance/medication-induced depressive disorder.
E. Persistent depressive disorder (dysthymia) and multiple sclerosis.

Correct Answer: C. Depressive disorder due to another medical condition.

Explanation: The essential feature of depressive disorder due to another medical condition is a prominent and persistent period of depressed mood or markedly diminished interest or pleasure in all, or almost all, activities that predominates in the clinical picture and that is thought to be related to the direct physiological effects of another medical condition. In determining whether the mood disturbance is due to another medical condition, the clinician must first establish the presence of such a condition. Furthermore, the clinician must establish that the mood disturbance is etiologically related to the other medical condition through a physiological mechanism. A careful and comprehensive assessment of multiple factors is necessary to make this judgment.

24—Depressive Disorder Due to Another Medical Condition / Diagnostic Features (p. 181)

25. An 18-year-old college student, recently arrived in the United States from Beijing, complains to her gynecologist of irritability, problems with her roommates, increased appetite, feeling bloated, and feeling depressed for 3–4 days prior to the onset of menses. She reports that these symptoms have been present since she reached menarche at age 12 (although she has never kept a mood log). The gynecologist calls you for a consultation about the correct diagnosis, because she is as yet unfamiliar with the new DSM-5 diagnostic criteria. What is your response?

    A. The patient has premenstrual syndrome because she does not meet criteria for premenstrual dysphoric disorder.
    B. The patient would qualify for a provisional diagnosis of premenstrual dysphoric disorder; however, the diagnosis does not exist in DSM-5.
    C. The patient would qualify for a provisional diagnosis of premenstrual dysphoric disorder.
    D. The patient would qualify for a provisional diagnosis of premenstrual dysphoric disorder if the diagnosis had been validated in Asian women.
    E. The patient has no DSM-5 diagnosis.

    Correct Answer: C. The patient would qualify for a provisional diagnosis of premenstrual dysphoric disorder.

Explanation: Premenstrual dysphoric disorder is not a culture-bound syndrome and has been observed in individuals in the United States, Europe, India, and Asia. It is unclear as to whether rates differ by race.

The essential features of premenstrual dysphoric disorder are the expression of mood lability, irritability, dysphoria, and anxiety symptoms that occur repeatedly during the premenstrual phase of the cycle and remit around the onset of menses or shortly thereafter. These symptoms may be accompanied by behavioral and physical symptoms. Symptoms must have occurred in most of the menstrual cycles during the past year and must have an adverse effect on work or social functioning.

Typically, symptoms peak around the time of the onset of menses. While the core symptoms include mood and anxiety symptoms, behavioral and somatic symptoms commonly also occur. In order to confirm a provisional diagnosis, daily prospective symptom ratings are required for at least two symptomatic cycles.

25—Premenstrual Dysphoric Disorder / Diagnostic Features; Culture-Related Diagnostic Issues (pp. 172–173)

26. What is the appropriate method of confirming a diagnosis of premenstrual dysphoric disorder?

    A. Laboratory tests.
    B. Family history.
    C. Neuropsychological testing.
    D. Two or more months of prospective symptom ratings on validated scales.
    E. One month of scoring high on the Daily Rating of Severity of Problems or 1 month of scoring high on the Visual Analogue Scales for Premenstrual Mood Symptoms.

Correct Answer: D. Two or more months of prospective symptom ratings on validated scales.

Explanation: The diagnosis of premenstrual dysphoric disorder is appropriately confirmed by 2 months of prospective symptom ratings. (Note: The diagnosis may be made provisionally prior to this confirmation.) A number of scales, including the Daily Rating of Severity of Problems and the Visual Analogue Scales for Premenstrual Mood Symptoms, have undergone validation and are commonly used in clinical trials for premenstrual dysphoric disorder. The Premenstrual Tension Syndrome Rating Scale has a self-report and an observer version, both of which have been validated and used widely to measure illness severity in women who have premenstrual dysphoric disorder.

26—Premenstrual Dysphoric Disorder / Diagnostic Markers (pp. 173–174)

27. A 29-year-old woman complains of sad mood every month in anticipation of her very painful menses. The pain begins with the start of her flow and continues for several days. She does not experience pain during other times of the month. She has tried a variety of treatments, none of which have given her relief. What is the appropriate diagnosis?

 A. Premenstrual dysphoric disorder.
 B. Premenstrual syndrome.
 C. Dysmenorrhea.
 D. Factitious disorder.
 E. Persistent depressive disorder (dysthymia).

Correct Answer: C. Dysmenorrhea.

Explanation: Dysmenorrhea is a syndrome of painful menses, but this is distinct from a syndrome characterized by affective changes. Symptoms of dysmenorrhea begin with the onset of menses, whereas symptoms of premenstrual dysphoric disorder, by definition, begin before the onset of menses, even if they linger into the first few days of menses.

27—Premenstrual Dysphoric Disorder / Differential Diagnosis (p. 174)

28. Which of the following symptoms must be present for a woman to meet criteria for premenstrual dysphoric disorder?

 A. Marked affective lability.
 B. Decreased interest in usual activities.
 C. Physical symptoms such as breast tenderness.
 D. Marked change in appetite.
 E. A sense of feeling overwhelmed or out of control.

Correct Answer: A. Marked affective lability.

Explanation: Of the 11 symptoms in the premenstrual dysphoric disorder diagnostic criteria, patients must have a total of at least 5 symptoms. One of the 5 must be one of the following symptoms: 1) marked affective lability; 2) marked irritability or anger or increased interpersonal conflicts; 3) marked depressed mood, feelings of hopelessness, or self-deprecating thoughts; 4) marked anxiety, tension, and/or feelings of being keyed up or on edge.

28—Premenstrual Dysphoric Disorder / diagnostic criteria (pp. 171–172)

29. A 23-year-old woman reports that during every menstrual cycle she experiences breast swelling, bloating, hypersomnia, an increased craving for sweets, poor concentration, and a feeling that she cannot handle her normal responsibilities. She notes that she also feels somewhat more sensitive emotionally and may become tearful when hearing a sad story. She takes no oral medication but

does use a drospirenone/ethinyl estradiol patch. What diagnosis best fits this clinical picture?

A. Premenstrual dysphoric disorder (PMDD).
B. Dysthymia.
C. Dysmenorrhea.
D. Premenstrual syndrome.
E. Substance/medication-induced depressive disorder.

Correct Answer: D. Premenstrual syndrome.

Explanation: Premenstrual syndrome differs from PMDD in that a minimum of five symptoms is not required and there is no stipulation of affective symptoms for individuals who suffer from premenstrual syndrome. This condition may be more common than PMDD, although the estimated prevalence of premenstrual syndrome varies. Premenstrual syndrome shares with PMDD the feature of symptom expression during the premenstrual phase of the menstrual cycle, but it is generally considered to be less severe than PMDD. Individuals who experience physical or behavioral symptoms in the premenstruum, without the required affective symptoms, likely meet criteria for premenstrual syndrome and not for PMDD.

29—Premenstrual Dysphoric Disorder / Differential Diagnosis (p. 174)

30. A 31-year-old woman with no history of mood symptoms reports that she experiences distressing mood lability and irritability starting about 4 days before the onset of menses. She feels "on edge," cannot concentrate, has little enjoyment from any of her activities, and experiences bloating and swelling of her breasts. The patient reports that these symptoms started 6 months ago when she began taking oral contraceptives for the first time. If she stops the oral contraceptives and her symptoms remit, what would the diagnosis be?

A. Premenstrual dysphoric disorder.
B. Dysthymia.
C. Major depressive episode.
D. Substance/medication-induced depressive disorder.
E. Premenstrual syndrome.

Correct Answer: D. Substance/medication-induced depressive disorder.

Explanation: If the woman stops the hormones and her symptoms disappear, this is consistent with substance/medication-induced depressive disorder. Some women who present with moderate to severe premenstrual symptoms may be using hormonal contraceptives. If such symptoms occur after initiation of exogenous hormone use, the symptoms may be due to the use of hormones rather than the underlying condition of premenstrual dysphoric disorder.

30—Premenstrual Dysphoric Disorder / Differential Diagnosis (pp. 174–175)

31. A 45-year-old man is admitted to the hospital with profound hypothyroidism. He is depressed but does not meet full criteria for major depressive disorder (MDD), the diagnosis given to him by his internist. The patient has no prior history of a mood disorder, and all of the depressive symptoms are temporally related to the hypothyroidism. Based on this information, you determine that a change in diagnosis—to depressive disorder due to another medical condition—is warranted, as well as a specifier to indicate that full criteria for MDD are not met. How would the full diagnosis be recorded?

   A. Hypothyroidism would be coded on Axis III in DSM-5.
   B. There is no special coding procedure in DSM-5.
   C. Hypothyroidism would be recorded as the name of the "other medical condition" in the DSM-5 diagnosis.
   D. Medical disorders are not coded as part of a mental disorder diagnosis in DSM-5.
   E. A revision to DSM-5 is planned to deal with this issue.

Correct Answer: C. Hypothyroidism would be recorded as the name of the "other medical condition" in the DSM-5 diagnosis.

Explanation: In recording a diagnosis of depressive disorder due to another medical condition, the name of the other medical condition is inserted in the mental disorder diagnosis (i.e., "depressive disorder due to hypothyroidism"). In addition, the other medical condition should be coded and listed separately immediately before the depressive disorder due to the medical condition. In this vignette, the full coding would be "244.9 [E03.9] hypothyroidism; 293.83 [F06.31] depressive disorder due to hypothyroidism, with depressive features." (The "with depressive features" specifier denotes that full criteria are not met for a major depressive episode.) There is no longer an Axis III in DSM-5.

31—Depressive Disorder Due to Another Medical Condition / diagnostic criteria (pp. 180–181)